THE **ART** AND **SCIENCE** OF TEACHING **ORIENTATION AND MOBILITY** TO PERSONS WITH VISUAL IMPAIRMENTS

William H. Jacobson, Ed.D.

PRESS

New York

The Art and Science of Teaching **Orientation and Mobility** *to Persons with Visual Impairments* is copyright © 1993 by

AFB Press
American Foundation for the Blind
15 West 16th Street, New York, NY 10011

97 96 95 94 93   5 4 3 2 1

Printed in the United States of America

Library of Congress Cataloging-in-Publication Data

Jacobson, William Henry.
    The art and science of teaching orientation and mobility to
persons with visual impairments / William H. Jacobson.
        p.   cm.
    Includes bibliographical references and index.
    ISBN 0-89128-245-9 (acid-free paper)
    1. Blind--Orientation and mobility--Study and teaching.   2. Blind-
-Rehabilitation--Study and teaching.   3. Space perception--Study and
teaching.
HV1758.J33 1993   93-21944
371.91 ' 1--dc20   CIP

Illustrations: Bonnie R. Jacobson
Photographs: William H. Jacobson; Darick Wright *(About the Author, p. 200)*

The mission of the American Foundation for the Blind (AFB) is to enable persons who are blind or visually impaired to achieve equality of access and opportunity that will ensure freedom of choice in their lives.

It is the policy of the American Foundation for the Blind to use in the first printing of its books acid-free paper that meets the ANSI Z39.48 Standard. The infinity symbol that appears above indicates that the paper in this printing meets that standard.

For Bon

Contents

Foreword

The ability to move about and travel safely and without assistance is one of the cornerstones of independence for people who are blind or visually impaired. For this reason, the profession of orientation and mobility (O&M) is an essential part of the blindness field, and noteworthy additions to the literature on O&M are important contributions to the field overall.

The Art and Science of Teaching Orientation and Mobility to Persons with Visual Impairments is such an addition. More than an outlining of the steps involved in various techniques, this new resource provides O&M instructors and assistants with an abundance of information on how to offer O&M instruction in an effective, creative, and individualized way. However, rehabilitation teachers and educators will also find that the first part of the book can be used by them as a text presenting explanations and strategies that they can use for reference purposes and that will help them make a maximum impact with clients. We at AFB Press are delighted to introduce the field to this important new work, a valuable tool that can be used in a variety of ways by a wide range of blindness professionals.

Carl R. Augusto
President and Executive Director
American Foundation for the Blind

Acknowledgments

One does not undertake a book of this sort alone. I wish to thank many individuals who, throughout the years, have provided me with the encouragement, support, and confidence to write this book. I especially want to express my indebtedness to my instructors at Boston College, Bill Walkowiak, Bob Smith, and Jack Burke; to Hugo Vigoroso, for providing me with the ability to analyze a task or problem; and to the late John Minor, who was my first mentor and gave me the confidence to bare my soul to my colleagues and to stick by my principles.

I must recognize my students and clients with visual impairments in Atlanta, Georgia, and Albany, New York, who probably taught me more about teaching than I taught them about mobility. Likewise, I am grateful to my more than 200 graduate orientation and mobility (O&M) students, who reconfirmed through their teachings that all the skills and techniques described here, although different in many minor and significant ways from the heretofore "accepted" practices, do, in fact, work.

More specifically, I thank the following students for reviewing the draft chapters associated with the techniques and using the skills during their blindfold, student teaching, and internship experiences to ensure that what I was describing made sense in written form: Kate Buck, Chuck Canterbury, John Carper, Susan Carper, Gwen Dina, Susan Flanders, Margie Flinton, Sherrie Frisbie, Lynn Gautreaux, Ron Halsell, Teresa Johnson, Ronee Krakowiak, Michelle Kregel, Ami Leberman, Bill McGeachy, David McMahon, Mary Ann Morrow, Jim Mullis, Sara Noel, Jeff Peach, Patricia Pokorny, Linda Starner, Diane Taylor, Sandy Weeks, and Michael Yamada. Also, I thank my graduate assistant, Kim Carr, for her help in researching Chapter 2; Dr. Ravic Ringlaben, for his contributions to an understanding of behavioral management in Chapter 1; Darick Wright, for researching cane manufacturers and his invaluable assistance with creative O&M approaches in Chapter 11; Joan Simms, for help with the life skills curriculum in Chapter 11; and my students Phyllis Gunderman, Pamela Hudson, Vance Saucier, and Sharon Smith, for agreeing to appear in photographs for this book.

The following university colleagues have helped me in too many ways throughout the years to mention here, but must be acknowledged as well: my O&M faculty colleagues, Jim Liska, Mimi Marsh, Nora Griffin-Shirley, Michael Williams Bliss, and Darick Wright; my rehabilitation and vision colleagues, Drs. Larry Dickerson, Patricia Bussen Smith, Dan Head, and Cay Holbrook; Dr. Gene Campbell, dean of the College of Education at the University of Arkansas at Little

Rock; and Dr. Tom Smith, formerly my faculty adviser at the University of Arkansas, Fayetteville, during my doctoral studies.

I would like to thank Mary Ellen Mulholland, Natalie Hilzen, JoAnne Chernow, Kathleen M. Huebner, and all the AFB staff for their advice, encouragement, and support in the development of this text. They made my first creation as painless as is humanly possible.

Finally, and most important, I must thank my wife, Bonnie Reines Jacobson, who has supported and encouraged me throughout my professional career, through its peaks and valleys, and who provided the illustrations for the text. Without her, I would not be who I am today, and this text would not have been possible.

Introduction

With the establishment of the first university graduate education program in peripatology at Boston College in 1960, the profession of orientation and mobility (O&M) was formally born. Before then, O&M had been confined primarily to the training of blinded veterans through the Veterans Administration, where the inception of "foot orientors," as they were called, evolved through the direction of Dr. Richard Hoover during World War II. Over the ensuing decades, O&M personnel training programs spread throughout the country.

The professional literature developed in the 1970s, most auspiciously with the publication of *Orientation and Mobility Techniques: A Guide for the Practitioner* (Hill & Ponder, 1976). Until then, instructors developed their own manuals during their training programs. Since the Hill and Ponder text, there has been only one other widely accepted text, *Orientation and Mobility: Behavioral Objectives for Teaching Older Adventitiously Blind Individuals* (Allen, Griffith, & Shaw, 1977), which was designed to teach O&M to elderly persons who have visual impairments using a behavioral approach. In 1980, the only text on the theories of teaching O&M was published, *Foundations of Orientation and Mobility* (Welsh & Blasch, 1980). Although revision of the latter is being undertaken, no revisions of any of these texts have been made to date since their initial printings.

These texts have been the primary components of the professional literature in the field until the present volume. This text has been designed to appeal to a new generation of persons who are interested in and capable of teaching some or all the skills of O&M. The first five chapters will be helpful not only to aspiring O&M instructors, but to classroom teachers of children with visual impairments, special education teachers, rehabilitation teachers, physical therapists, occupational therapists, nurses, and aides to these professionals. These chapters describe an overview of the teaching of O&M skills by treating the student as an individual (Chapter 1); the principles underlining the development of the motor skills and concepts necessary for adequate O&M (Chapter 2); and the basic O&M skills of the sighted guide (Chapter 3), self-protection (Chapter 4), and diagonal cane techniques (Chapter 5). In addition, these chapters outline in detail how to select teaching environments, how to sequence lessons for an individualized approach to learning, the importance of finding and using landmarks and compass directions, and how to familiarize oneself to rooms in a building.

The remaining chapters address the skills, techniques, and issues that have direct relevance for the aspiring O&M instructor. How to travel through familiar and unfa-

xii THE ART AND SCIENCE OF TEACHING O&M

miliar indoor and outdoor environments is discussed at length in Chapters 6-9. Chapters 10-12 address special travel situations and issues that confront the O&M instructor on a daily basis. How the student uses escalators, elevators, and revolving doors; travels during adverse weather conditions; uses public transportation; and uses electronic travel aids and collapsible canes are subjects addressed in Chapter 10. In Chapter 11, creative teaching approaches are described, including such topics as small- and large-group seminars, safely teaching more than one student at a time, drop-off and solo lessons, and working with other professionals and family members. Professional issues such as the mobility code of ethics, client confidentiality, and continued lifelong learning and sharing of expertise are discussed in Chapter 12.

These chapters are meant to complement rather than supplant university training programs. Entire courses address the medical aspects of blindness and associated disabilities, the psychological aspects of blindness, and how to teach the methods skills. University students simulate being a student with a visual impairment under carefully controlled conditions and under the tutelage of a university faculty member or an experienced adjunct instructor and develop an empathic understanding of the special problems associated with learning travel skills. The students practice teaching the skills to each other before teaching them to actual students with visual impairments during their student teaching or internships. These educational programs last upwards of a year or longer.

Other interested persons are therefore discouraged from attempting to implement any of these techniques or procedures. Unless one is willing to assume the risks and potential liability associated with teaching these skills, the instruction of these techniques should be left to the professionally trained O&M instructor.

THE POPULATION SERVED BY THIS TEXT

This text describes the techniques and procedures used to teach O&M to persons with severe visual impairments or who are totally blind. It does not address work with individuals who have additional impairments because it is meant to offer a foundation from which techniques and procedures can be adapted and modified for all other individuals. Instructors must use the information garnered from this text judiciously, along with their university training, to work with the various populations they will encounter during the course of their careers. Since the text is meant to supplement university courses on theory and methods, it is expected that university programs will supplement the information presented herein with additional courses, seminars, and workshops. The material presented in Chapter 2, for instance, could constitute an entire university course or several courses. It merely highlights those issues and concerns related to understanding concepts; it does not attempt to instruct the student in how to teach the concepts, which is best left to the university program through its academic courses and its student teaching and internship experiences.

Furthermore, the text is designed to help one instruct either children or adults, irrespective of age, using different approaches. With some children, the instructor may break up the lesson into several components to ensure continued interest and, through creative lesson planning that promotes student-directed learning in real-life situations, stimulate the students' motivation to learn and use the mobility skills. With elderly students, the instructor may also break up the lesson to allow the student to rest. The goals and objectives should be developed in conjunction with each student's interests.

The O&M program matches the student's age, gender, intelligence level, and particular needs. For example, very young students may not be taught how to cross streets until they are at the appropriate age—even if they have the skills to do so, although some instructors believe it is important to give very young students a slight "edge" on their sighted peers by teaching them skills such as this at an earlier-than-normal age. In addition, instructors must be cognizant that teenage students of the opposite sex may develop a crush on them, particularly since they work so closely and intimately together. Furthermore, students who are cognitively challenged may not be expected to learn at the same rate and level of skills as those who are not, and so lessons may be broken down into smaller components, skills may be practiced and drilled over longer periods, and lower levels of attainment may be accepted. Finally, some students may live and work in areas that may not necessitate their learning the entire range of skills presented here. For instance, one who lives and works in a farming community may never have the interest or the need to travel on subways or in large, downtown environments; therefore, traveling in rural areas, described in Chapter 9, may constitute the student's entire mobility program.

HOW TO USE THIS TEXT

This text was designed sequentially to take the university O&M student through an O&M program as if he or she were an individual with a visual impairment. The skills presented here are the foundations on which to build an individualized O&M program for each student or client. The term *student*, used throughout the text, refers to a learner of skills, rather than solely to a young person in school. Likewise, the term *instructor* refers to the teacher, specialist, or therapist who provides the instruction. To avoid the use of sexist language, in successive chapters, the gender description of each individual in the student-instructor team alternates between the instructor being a female or a male and the student being a male or a female, except when a general statement concerning students and instructors is being made, in which case the plural form is used.

There is no one right way to teach O&M. If one is looking for a "cookbook" approach to learning O&M, this text will be a disappointment. Each skill is presented in a paragraph format that introduces the skill, describes the sequential procedures in accomplishing the skill, and then discusses additional considerations when teaching the skill. The suggested sequence is the one that the profession has generally agreed is acceptable for many students. However, in some instances it may be more appropriate to introduce a skill or concept at a different time or in a different way. For example, some students who are being taught in their home environments may, out of necessity, have to learn cane skills quickly and then learn more of the basic mobility skills later.

Each skill or procedure may be thought of as a mini-unit that must be broken down into its smallest parts, learned, practiced, and drilled until it can be replicated at will whenever necessary. Those who simulate persons with visual impairments through blindfold training to become O&M instructors will discover that they will not have acquired the same skills as have their students. Their goal, in using this text, is to understand the underlying principles and procedures needed to become safe and efficient travelers with visual impairments. As one will see, the only true way to get to Carnegie Hall is to practice, practice, practice!

Illustrations

Unit One

BASIC INDOOR ORIENTATION AND MOBILITY SKILLS: PREDICATES TO INDEPENDENT MOBILITY

Chapters in this first unit describe how persons with visual impairments understand and organize the space around them. This unit is especially designed for many types of instructors. Those who want to be orientation and mobility (O&M) specialists will find it especially helpful in understanding the role that the various senses play in the orientation process and the beginning techniques required to navigate safely through a familiar, indoor environment. Classroom teachers and rehabilitation teachers will learn how to teach basic O&M skills to their students and clients. Other professionals, such as nurses, physical therapists, occupational therapists, and low vision specialists, will find these theories and techniques useful in helping their patients with visual impairments learn to negotiate their immediate indoor surroundings. Nurse's aides, ward attendants, and mobility assistants will find these chapters useful in complementing the lessons taught by the foregoing professionals. Although some of these paraprofessionals may initiate instruction, it is recommended that they reinforce, practice, and drill students or clients with visual impairments on these techniques after the initial lessons have been taught by professionals. Finally, parents and other relatives will discover the reasons why the mobility process evolves as it does and learn the basic techniques necessary in beginning the mobility learning process.

Chapter 1 introduces the various professionals who are involved in the mobility process and the approach of instructing behaviors in a prescribed manner. Chapter 2 presents the concepts of body imagery, motor functioning, and environmental awareness; explains the roles that the remaining senses play in maintaining or regaining one's orientation in space; and discusses the role of the O&M instructor in assessing a student's understanding of various concepts and how to teach concepts that are found to be lacking.

Chapter 3 describes the techniques and procedures used to aid the student in walking with sighted assistance. This is the first formal step in the O&M teaching process and begins the development of trust and rapport between the student and the instructor. The chapter also discusses how to sequence the lessons, choose environments for the lessons, and find and use landmarks and clues for orientation and special situations that may occur while using the sighted guide procedures.

After students have begun to master the sighted guide procedures, they may be ready to learn how to walk into open spaces indoors while protecting themselves from protruding obstacles and hazards. They should begin to explore the environment in a systematic way. Chapter 4 describes in detail the basic self-protection techniques and considerations for more effective teaching, including sequencing lessons and choosing an appropriate environment for lessons, special teaching techniques, route patterns, and numbering systems. The techniques and skills in Chapter 5 may be taught by O&M specialists or others interested in helping their students or clients to acquire basic skills. Classroom teachers, rehabilitation teachers, physical therapists, occupational therapists, and nurses will find the descriptions of the diagonal cane technique and the room-familiarization procedures especially helpful in orienting their students or clients to their homes, classrooms, or agencies. However, it is the role of the O&M instructor to prescribe and obtain the appropriate long cane for the student.

1

Teaching Orientation and Mobility

In this chapter, you will learn the roles that various professionals play in helping students with visual impairments learn orientation and mobility (O&M). Who are the O&M specialists, and what training do they receive? Who are the other specialists, and what are their roles in this process? How does the O&M instructor help others change previously learned ways of doing things so they can accomplish their goals more effectively?

WHAT IS O&M?

Orientation is the ability to use one's remaining senses to understand one's location in the environment at any given time. *Mobility* is the capacity or facility of movement. *Orientation and mobility* may be defined, then, as the teaching of the concepts, skills, and techniques necessary for a person with a visual impairment to travel safely, efficiently, and gracefully through any environment and under all environmental conditions and situations. O&M instructors are individuals who are formally educated to help persons with visual impairments attain their O&M goals. Certified O&M specialists meet minimal competencies defined and endorsed by Division IX (Orientation and Mobility) of the international professional association, the Association for Education and Rehabilitation of the Blind and Visually Impaired (AER). Initially, these competencies are gained through the completion of approved university training programs in O&M. Every five years, certified mobility specialists must show proof of having taught a prescribed number of hours of O&M and of having completed a prescribed number of continuing education units. Some states require additional state certification or endorsements for those who wish to teach O&M in such areas as teaching children with general special education needs, teaching children with visual impairments, and specifically teaching O&M. In some instances, potential instructors must show proof of having completed appro-

priate university course work or must take written competency tests in these subject areas.

Other professionals who teach or reinforce certain basic skills include the classroom teacher, the rehabilitation teacher, the physical therapist, the occupational
therapist, the nurse, and the low vision specialist (a teacher who has been specially
trained in low vision skills or an optometrist or an ophthalmologist who specializes
in low vision). Still others, such as O&M assistants, teaching assistants, and nursing
aides, provide practice and drill in certain techniques or procedures.

OVERVIEW OF O&M INSTRUCTION: A HOLISTIC APPROACH

The teaching of O&M skills is as much an art as it is a science. Knowing how and
when to combine teaching orientation skills and mobility skills is the core of the
process. When to help or intervene if the student becomes disoriented and when to
let the student work through the problem are dilemmas that the instructor confronts in each lesson. Thus, the instructor must develop individualized programs
that not only teach the skills but help students build confidence in their travel abilities so they can take responsibility for their actions and accept the consequences of
their decisions. Lessons are taught in the home community, when possible, and are
developed to meet the special needs of each student. If it is not feasible to do so,
lessons are designed to represent the students' home areas as closely as possible, so
the students can transfer what they have learned to that environment. Additional
lessons are designed to help some students travel in places with which they are not
familiar.

The O&M process begins with the seemingly simple step of learning to walk
with a sighted guide. By using sighted assistance, the students not only begin to
accept help from others when a situation warrants it, but learn that they have control over a situation in that they can ask appropriate questions about the immediate
area they are walking through so they can come back to the area by themselves at
another time. Likewise, they can discontinue help if they are not satisfied with it.
As the sequence outlined in Chapters 3-10 evolves, students learn to travel independently (or interdependently) to or through various types of environments. As
they gain experience and exposure to these situations, they develop the necessary
skills to take the responsibility for their actions, to solve problems when they
become disoriented, and to become reoriented with little or no help from others.

The most difficult aspect of teaching these skills is to remember that students
are experiencing a multitude of other problems in their daily lives that may affect
how they learn the skills. By putting themselves in the students' shoes, so to speak,
instructors may gain a better understanding of why students may be having difficulty with instruction. Instructors must remember that the teaching of orientation
skills together with mobility skills is not necessarily a concurrent process. Although
the two skills go hand in hand, they must first be taught in isolation before students

can integrate them and use them simultaneously. For example, in teaching a particular skill, such as the two-point-touch cane technique (Chapter 6), the instructor concentrates on the mechanics of how that skill is accomplished. The student practices swinging the cane and walking in step and in rhythm over and over again until the skill is learned or overlearned. Then the instructor introduces an orientation skill or skills. For instance, a student may be taught not only to walk down a hallway while using the appropriate two-point-touch technique, but to maintain compass directions and identify landmarks. As the instructor quizzes the student on these orientation skills, she may notice that his cane skills have become deficient. Is it because he really did not learn the cane skills, or is it because he cannot concentrate on both of them simultaneously? It is probably the latter. It takes much time to engrain both a motor skill and a cognitive skill. Therefore, the instructor's expectations must be different at the beginning and end of a unit of instruction. When the student can integrate the motor skill with the cognitive skill and can demonstrate that he has done so in a novel situation, the instructor can safely say that the student has learned the particular technique. In sum, the instructor must view not only the student, but the teaching of O&M, in a holistic manner.

ROLES OF THE O&M INSTRUCTOR AND OTHERS

The O&M instructor has the primary role in providing mobility instruction in the traditional sense. However, others also have major responsibilities in helping the student to learn and use these skills. Parents of children with visual impairments, especially those of very young children, play a direct and influential role in helping their infants and toddlers acquire basic mobility skills because they are with their children most of the time. Since they must be knowledgeable about the skills that need to be reinforced and taught, the O&M instructor shows them how and what to teach by modeling the process with the children. With older children, the instructor becomes the primary teacher and the parents monitor some techniques and provide encouragement, support, and follow-up training. Other significant family members and friends also follow up on mobility instruction after they have met with and been counseled by the O&M instructor on a regular basis.

In the schools, the classroom teacher, vision consultant, teacher's aide, and even a student's peers all reinforce the skills the student has acquired. Sometimes the teacher and aide provide primary instruction of basic mobility skills (see Chapters 1-5) if time and situations permit.

In agencies, rehabilitation teachers and rehabilitation counselors may provide basic skills training, especially if they work in the students' home settings, or they may provide reinforcement by encouraging their students to use the skills they learned during mobility lessons. Family members are encouraged to reinforce the use of skills and techniques that have been learned by students, especially when the students are at home. Mobility assistants, especially trained by an O&M

instructor and certified as such by AER, provide training in basic skills and follow-up instruction in basic skills training taught by the O&M instructor.

THE ROAD TO INTERDEPENDENCE: GUIDELINES FOR THE INSTRUCTOR

O&M lessons for both adults and children should always be success oriented. The overall concepts or goals of the lesson should be broken down into smaller components at first and then built upon as these components are mastered. The environment in which one works should be nonthreatening and easily controllable at first and then become more complex and less controlled as skills are learned and the lessons progress, by which time the student should be prepared to handle such conditions. However, if the student has not yet experienced a situation or learned a particular technique or procedure, the instructor should not expect him to be able to handle it effectively at first. When the student masters the situation or technique, the instructor places more responsibility on him for his actions and reactions. By the end of a unit (or mobility program, for that matter), the student should be responsible for his own actions and accountable for them. Both the student and instructor should be so comfortable with the skills the student has learned that he can be expected to travel to various destinations without the instructor observing and intervening. Solo lessons, explained in Chapter 11 in greater detail, are culminating experiences for both the student and instructor that prove that the student has confidence in his travel skills and can travel independently. To reach this end, children often require a developmental approach to learning. They need to learn appropriate motor and conceptual skills when they are ready to do so and to learn them in real-life situations. Each successive skill builds on the mastery of lesser skills. Thus, learning about oneself (body imagery) leads to an understanding of objects in space, which, in turn, leads to an understanding of space and its relationship to the individual. However, many children who do not learn these concepts initially in sequence learn many of the concepts later in life.

Adult learners who lost their vision later in life need to have their access to the environment restored, whereas those who were born with a visual impairment may need to learn concepts they did not learn previously. The approach to their training is less direct than the approach to training children.

Each learner is an individual and must be treated as such. Categorizing a student by intellectual level, eye condition, or other impairments prompts a connotation that may be simplistic or even erroneous. Many persons, regardless of their intellectual level or additional impairments, may become excellent travelers. On the other hand, many individuals who are highly intelligent may not learn the necessary travel skills because of their overriding fear of travel.

But what does it mean to be an interdependent as opposed to an independent traveler? Does it mean doing everything by oneself without any help from anyone else? Or does it mean knowing one's limitations and seeking and using assistance from others as the situations warrant? None of us lives in a vacuum. We are constantly asking others for assistance. To find a store in an unfamiliar neighborhood, we telephone the store and ask for directions; to find a particular street if we are lost in a section of a city, we stop at a gas station to ask for help. We use road maps to travel between cities and states. Knowing how to rely on or gain help from others when it is needed, then, is the real sign of independence.

Along the road to interdependence, instructors must ensure the safety of their students. The road is fraught with potential dangers. Bumping into partially opened doors, tripping down stairs or off curbs or into manholes, or stepping into oncoming traffic are all potential hazards that O&M instructors are trained to expect and to teach students how to avoid or minimize. The rapport that instructors develop with their students depends on their trust of each other throughout the program. Without this basic trust, instructors and students cannot achieve their ultimate goals. Students must know that their instructors will not place them in potentially harmful situations that they are not prepared to handle.

BEHAVIORAL OBJECTIVES AND TASK ANALYSIS

Teaching simple or complex O&M skills to individuals can be a challenge to any instructor. The use of applied behavior analysis can provide the instructor with a means to bring about necessary and lasting changes in students' behavior and skills.

Applied behavior analysis involves viewing any "activity" of the student as a "behavior" that can be influenced to occur more often or less often. The entry level of a behavior, often referred to as baseline behavior, has generally not been influenced by a structured program or intervention. It is determined by observing and evaluating a student's initial skills. For example, during the initial assessment, the instructor observes that the student has not been taught the skills to walk with a sighted guide (Chapter 3), which may be called the entry level of the behavior. Any subsequent training to learn sighted guide skills would then be considered a behavioral change even though the student did not actually have a "behavior" in the traditional sense to be changed.

Deficient and Interfering Behaviors

Behaviors to be changed can be classified as deficient or interfering. Deficient skills or behaviors are new ones that need to be taught or those that need to be increased or improved so the individual does them more often or at a level of higher skill. These behaviors or skills are generally described in the teaching units as mobility skills. When learning the diagonal cane technique (Chapter 5), for instance, the student may at first not keep his hand and arm in the correct position. But over time and with much practice, the student is finally able to maintain the correct position, so that the "deficient" skill may be considered "learned."

Interfering behaviors are problem behaviors (like speaking when the instructor is speaking; banging a cane on the ground; or such blind manneristic behaviors as rocking back and forth and swaying one's head) that generally obstruct the learning of appropriate O&M behaviors. It may be important to reduce or eliminate these behaviors so the individual can learn or maintain the appropriate mobility skills. For instance, if a student sways his head, his ability to localize auditory cues may be impaired (Chapter 2), which, in turn, could impair the student's ability to gauge the precise direction of the flow of traffic and thus could compromise his ability to cross streets (Chapter 8).

Instructional Objectives

Often, instructors make the mistake of attempting only to reduce the interfering behaviors and assume that the appropriate skills will somehow evolve on their own. It is important to develop a plan that focuses on and teaches appropriate behaviors to replace the interfering ones. In evaluating students' needs, instructors must describe goals and objectives for their students specifically to ensure progress and to let students know exactly what they will be learning, so the students can focus their energies on acquiring the skills. Each student is an individual with different levels of skills and entry, deficient, and interfering behaviors and thus requires an individualized teaching plan and objectives.

After the instructor has identified the behaviors and skills that the student needs to learn or change, she develops appropriate end objectives for the student—behaviors or skills that the student will demonstrate at the conclusion of the instructional program. The instructor must carefully determine and define exactly what the student will do as a result of the proposed intervention. Behavioral objectives detail the conditions under which the behavior is presented (e.g., on a corner of a four-lane street), the behavior (e.g., walking while swinging the cane), and the criteria for acceptable performance. Statements indicating criteria should include components that address speed (e.g., in 10 seconds or less), accuracy (e.g., in a straight line), and mastery (e.g., on three successive occasions). One example of an appropriate behavioral objective may be this: "While walking down a hallway, the student will demonstrate the ability to maintain his hand at midline when using the two-point-touch cane technique on four out of five successive I-routes."

Task Analysis

The steps an instructor follows to move the student from baseline levels to the terminal objective can be clarified through the use of task analysis—the process by which a complex behavior is broken down into its simplest components and steps. All of us have learned complex behaviors like tying shoes and operating a computer by this process. The separate tasks involved in swinging a long cane using the two-point-touch cane technique (Chapter 6) may include what may be thought of as "prerequisite" skills and "procedural" tasks. In this case, *prerequisite skills* may include the ability to maintain an upright posture, to understand laterality (which arm and muscles will be used to swing the cane) and directionality (the cane position in front of the waist), to have fine motor control (to swing the cane), to have gross motor control (to walk in step and in rhythm), to have kinesthetic understanding (to swing the cane laterally to maintain a constant arc width), and to walk with an appropriate gait pattern. The *procedural tasks* are the actual steps in completing the process of swinging and walking with the cane, as described in detail in Chapter 6. Naturally, an individualized approach to teaching must be developed to help students develop these skills as they learn the mobility tasks. Students can learn higher-level skills without some prerequisite skills, but they might perform them at less-than-acceptable levels. The instructor must remember, however, that if the student cannot perform any of these skills, he must be taught to do so. These skills will not just magically occur.

Behavioral Links and Chains

An entire complex behavior can be thought of as a "chain," and the steps in presenting the behavior can be thought of as "links." The most complex behavior begins with the first link. Therefore, a separate behavioral objective is written for each link in the chain, and it is important that students demonstrate competence by meeting criteria on an objective (link) before instruction begins on the next objective (link). Chains can be taught "forward" or "backward." The forward-chain procedure can be applied to teach a complex skill, like swinging a long cane. The instructor begins by teaching link 1 (grasping the cane) and then proceeds to link 2 (extending the cane out from the body), and so on. Sometimes students become frustrated when they are taught using the forward-chain process because they recognize that they will not demonstrate the complete skill until they learn the last link.

A backward-chain procedure solves this problem by teaching the last link first (e.g., the last stretch of the route to the storefront). After the last link is learned, then the last two are introduced and learned, and so forth. In this approach, the complex behavior is always successfully completed during each instructional session. Although it may not be the typical way of learning or teaching, this procedure is a successful approach to teaching complex skills, especially to students with developmental disabilities who may not understand how they will get to the end product (the destination) after they have been taught each successive phase of the route for several weeks or months using the forward-chain approach.

Long-Term Goals

After the initial assessment, the instructor determines with the student the long-term goals and objectives that will be incorporated into the mobility program. These goals will be determined, in part, by the amount of time available for lessons. How long will each lesson be? How many sessions will there be each week and each month? For how many months or years will instruction be conducted? Children in schools generally have an advantage over adults in agencies in that they are taught for many years, whereas adults are constrained by the amount of rehabilitation funds available for much shorter periods, typically 6-12 weeks. Furthermore, adults' needs may change as their eye and other health conditions deteriorate (or improve) or their living and working conditions change.

Therefore, what may be viewed as long-term goals for adults may be viewed as short-term objectives for children.

A typical student who is totally blind with no other additional impairments and who receives instruction five days a week for an hour a day usually needs 150-200 hours over 12-18 months, depending upon his needs and previous experiences. Instruction dealing with indoor travel (Chapters 2-6) may take 30-60 hours to complete and sets the stage for the outdoor units. Each individual outdoor unit may then take progressively fewer and fewer hours to accomplish because each builds on the foundation of those that have preceded it.

Students who have additional impairments or other complications may take much longer to complete their programs. They may need additional time to learn and practice appropriate motor skills or additional exposure to travel areas to experience different situations. If the goals are limited, they will need less time. Some students may not need or want to travel in rural (or conversely, downtown) areas, so their programs will not include such units. One example of a long-term goal may be: "The student demonstrates the ability to travel in a downtown area by (1) using acceptable long cane skills while walking along sidewalks 100 percent of the time, (2) crossing streets in an acceptable manner 100 percent of the time, and (3) locating identifiable landmarks and stores 100 percent of the time." As one can see, the goals are broad in scope yet specific in outcomes.

Short-Term Objectives

After several long-term goals are developed, the instructor determines the short-term objectives and estimates the entire time it will take to complete them. She then backs up from the approximated ending date and divides the time into smaller units, either weekly or monthly, and develops short-term objectives that lead to the achievement of the long-term goals. These objectives can be further broken down into smaller objectives that are incorporated into the individual lesson plans. The weekly lesson plans, then, lead to the accomplishment of the weekly short-term objectives, which, in turn, leads to the eventual accomplishment of the long-term goals.

One example of a short-term objective may be as follows: "The student uses acceptable long cane skills to walk along a sidewalk by (1) maintaining the proper step, rhythm and arc height-width over 90 percent of each route, (2) walking around detected objects without touching them with his hand 100 percent of the time on each route, and (3) detecting each curb at every corner with the long cane 100 percent of the time on each route."

Each objective has criteria that are definable and measurable. Each criterion is directed at what the student will do and accomplish. Skills progress from the simple to achieve to the more complex. Lessons (or the objectives) are repeated as many times as are necessary to meet the criteria for each objective. The instructor may wish to develop a chart to note the number of trials (e.g., routes) and the number of times a particular behavior is exhibited. By using this behavioral approach, she can easily gauge the success or failure of a particular skill or lesson and adjust her teaching approach, if necessary, and compare the new approach to earlier approaches. If the new approach is successful, she can duplicate it in future lessons and share it with other instructors.

THE CONCEPT OF OVERLEARNING

As was mentioned earlier, motor skills must be broken down into their components and each component must be built on previous ones until the entire skill is achieved. To do so, the instructor analyzes the task involved, breaks it down into subtasks, and teaches the subcomponents one after the other until the student learns the whole task.

When an instructor is teaching a student to swing the cane using the two-point-touch cane technique, she builds each of the following aspects of the skill on the next to ensure that the student consistently detects curbs or stair drop-offs or obstacles in the path: (1) grasping the cane in a prescribed manner, (2) holding it at midline and waist height, and (3) swinging it so it sweeps to cover the widest part of one's body from side to side. When one is walking, the cane lightly touches down at the farthest point of the arc on either side of the body. As each foot touches the ground, the respective heel touches at the same time as the cane tip (in rhythm). Likewise, the cane tip touches down where the next foot placement approximately will be (in step).

The skill is made up of numerous fine motor and gross motor skills. Once analyzed, the skill is broken down into its component parts and is taught sequentially. If one part is not learned sufficiently, succeeding aspects of the technique will suffer accordingly. If the cane is improperly grasped, for example, the user will have difficulty with the fine motor skills of pushing it with the finger or wrist—without moving the entire arm or rotating the wrist. If the wrist rotates, the cane tip will come off the ground several inches or more, which will make it difficult or impossible for the user to detect curbs or other drop-off areas and may result in the person's tripping off curbs or stairs and injuring himself.

The instructor isolates and teaches the first skill—grasping the cane. Once the student feels comfortable grasping the cane, the instructor then introduces the hand position in relation to the student's midline and waist height. Facing the student, she may gently hold the student's wrist to place it in the correct position until she no longer feels resistance from the student. As the student pushes the cane from side to side, the instructor lets him tap the insides of her feet with the cane tip; her feet are placed to approximate the widest part of the arc width of the cane arc. As the student gains proficiency, he will lightly touch the instructor's feet with the cane tip and his wrist will not press against the instructor's hand. After the student has mastered these skills, the instructor backs away from him and provides verbal feedback as he swings the cane.

To ensure that the student has indeed learned the motor skill, the instructor helps him to overlearn it. That is, she provides time for him to demonstrate proficiency beyond her normal expectations. For example, if the instructor believes that the student will have demonstrated the proper technique in step and in rhythm by being able to walk down a corridor ten times without going out of step or out of rhythm, she then may require him to do so an additional five times. This concentration, practice, and drill help the student overlearn the concept and thus help him to develop the kinesthetic feeling necessary to reproduce the skill whenever necessary.

The concept of overlearning is important for any motor skill. If the skill is not overlearned, the student will probably not be able to reproduce it whenever he needs to, which is why many students with visual impairments hold their hands off to their dominant sides, which causes them to lose forward coverage on their nondominant side and places them in jeopardy of falling off curbs or stairs with the nondominant foot (Croce & Jacobson, 1986).

Motor skills, therefore, are the predicates to efficient mobility. But without proper orientation skills, one's mobility will be limited. In the next several chapters in this unit, you will learn how to develop initial sequential mobility skills while introducing the student to proper orientation skills. As you shall see, the student may have great difficulty concentrating on one while trying to accomplish the other. Motor skills need to become ingrained before students can be expected to concentrate on higher-level orientation skills. The road to independence guides the student to a delicate balance between the two.

2

Maintaining One's Orientation in Space

Vision plays an important role in the way we perceive and understand our environment. Through the use of vision, we process in our memories images of the world around us to monitor how we must move through space efficiently, effortlessly, and gracefully. If our visual system becomes impaired, we must learn new ways to use our sensory impressions to modify and adapt our movements to compensate for this new way of perceiving the people and objects in our environment.

Individuals who have lost their vision partially or totally must compensate by learning to use their remaining senses in new and different ways. This chapter explores what it means to adapt to the world without sight or with impaired vision. You will learn that we all must first understand our bodies and how they function to comprehend the complex arrangements of the objects in the spaces about us and that as we move about the environment, the spatial relationships of these objects change in relation to our positions. People who cannot visualize themselves with some consistency in these ever-changing environments will function in limited or different ways.

MOTOR FUNCTIONING

To have a desire to move, an individual must receive sensory impressions. Otherwise, movements are merely random and do not become purposeful. Children who are born blind or with a visual impairment do not have ways to observe and imitate those who move around them. Often, they develop in different but slower ways than do children who have an intact visual system. At critical stages of motor development, many children who are visually impaired exhibit developmental lags in learning to creep, crawl, kneel, stand, walk, hop, skip, and jump that may last for one to several months or for much longer periods (Fraiberg, Smith, & Adelson, 1969).

Naturally, the longer the lag is allowed to continue, the further behind motorically the children will be in relation to their peers. But it is possible to intervene during these developmental lags to prod the children to the next stage of motor development. The first step in overcoming a motor deficit is to understand how the body and body parts function—that is, to have good body imagery. Without good body imagery, one has difficulty making efficient use of the incoming sensory impressions to move with understanding and purpose through the environment.

BODY IMAGERY

Body imagery may be involuntary or voluntary. Although involuntary body imagery, which includes dreams, hallucinations, and visual memories, may serve a purpose in the course of one's life, it is not useful for a discussion of movement through space, especially for those who have never seen. However, voluntary imagery, which includes memory, imagination, awareness of the environment, everyday life experiences, problem solving, anticipating the future, and feeling secure about oneself in the environment, is helpful in understanding and relating to one's environment.

In terms of this discussion, all people must develop a mental image of themselves to imagine that they are standing in, walking through, and interacting with the environment. This image becomes the focal point about which all future impressions are made. Persons with a visual impairment can achieve this image by remembering past movements and encounters with objects and people in various situations. By touching, tasting, smelling, and listening to the sensory impressions around them, they can develop a positive and consistent self-image and learn about the environment in meaningful ways—even without the use of vision. Over time, these perceptions and impressions dictate how all people respond to future situations and conditions. Therefore, it is important to explore the environment to learn how one belongs in it.

Children with visual impairments begin (as do all children) by learning about themselves. They must understand how their body parts relate to and interact with each other. They must be able to identify not only their individual body parts, but their left arm and right leg, left thigh and right calf, or upper arm and lower leg, for example. Eventually, they should be able to recognize someone else's right arm or leg (or other body parts) so they can visualize themselves in different spatial positions. How well they understand the ramifications of positioning when they turn their bodies ever so slightly (or dramatically) will dictate their reactions to and interactions with the people and objects they encounter. The more discretely they can identify and understand their body parts and their functioning, the better they will understand the consequences of their actions and positions in the space about them.

Finally, to understand how they move through the environment, visually impaired children must know how their arms and legs rotate and bend; how their feet become planted on the ground; and how they can push off differently for purposeful movements like walking, running, and jumping. Because they cannot merely watch others doing these skills, they must be shown how to do them. Since they have never seen others move their body parts, each limb and joint may have to be manipulated into the correct position and movement. They may have to be given lots of encouragement and time to learn these skills in a variety of different ways.

Children or adults who experience visual impairments later in life (that is, who are adventitiously visually impaired) have different problems. If they have adequate visual memories from which to draw, they must learn when to use them and when to ignore them and use other pieces of information to help them become oriented. Often, they have other difficulties to overcome that usually revolve around coping with their vision loss, especially coping with a different set of sensory impressions. Most sighted people have learned how their body parts function and enable them to interact with the environment and how to use their vision to compensate for any shortcomings in conceptualization. That is, if they have doubts about how they should swing their arms when they walk, they need only observe others walking. It is irrelevant whether they truly understand the concept of purposeful arm swinging so long as they can adequately mimic the movements. However, without visual input, people cannot simply look to see how they should be moving their limbs or where they are going. Hence, people who are adventitiously visually impaired quickly realize that they must literally learn to walk all over again. Often, this is the biggest obstacle to achieving independence from or interdependence with others.

MOTOR CONTROL, STRENGTH, AND ENDURANCE

Motor skills are learned in three stages. In the first stage, skills are consciously executed and are dependent on cognition, or understanding. Movement is controlled by automatic responses from the various sensory systems—vision, hearing, and touch. The infant or child with a visual impairment responds to sensory impressions by reaching out for the audible mobile overhanging the crib or by trying to grasp the rattle placed on her stomach, for example. If the object presented crosses over the *midline*, or the center of the body, the movement of reaching for it may cause the infant to roll over from her back to her stomach. In this position, the infant can learn to creep and crawl to move about the immediate space. Therefore, parents are encouraged to find ways to coax an infant to reach for objects across her midline so she will learn to roll over onto her stomach.

Learning How to Explore

After the infant has learned to initiate movements, she enters the second stage of motor skill development. She must practice the movements and learn to detect errors in them and to control the motor acts effectively. In short, she must move to explore and explore to move. But, without visual feedback, the infant will not know if she is moving efficiently or purposefully. Thus, her parents and siblings will have to teach her. They can provide safe areas in which to explore space and the encouragement and incentives to move about. At first, a playpen filled with toys to touch, twist, turn, and taste is the safe haven for the infant with a visual impairment. Later, the floor of her room and then of other rooms in the house or apartment can be explored. The infant is encouraged to move about; to creep and crawl; to grab onto and stand up; and, eventually, to stand up unsupported and walk. In this process she will inevitably bump her head on a table or chair or fall down and become bruised. But without these experiences, she will not understand the consequences of her movements.

In the third stage, the child subconsciously initiates movement and develops motivation and understanding. She wishes to explore a place, touch something, or go somewhere. Cognition supersedes the motor movements. She no longer thinks about how to move her limbs to complete the motor skills. The motor skills are accomplished sufficiently to reach the purported objective.

To reach the third stage of any motor skill, the child (or adult) must be shown how to perform the skill correctly and be given ample opportunity to practice the skill until it is performed subconsciously whenever it is needed. Everyone—with or without a visual impairment—learns a motor skill this way. The difference is in how the skill is executed and practiced.

Modeling Motor Skills

Motor skills must be demonstrated, and the skills must be broken down into smaller units. The person must be allowed to repeat the smaller movements of the motor skill and add them together to produce the overall skill. Once she can do so, she achieves a kinesthetic understanding of the skill. That is, once the skill becomes ingrained, it can be replicated over and over at will. This kinesthetic understanding is also called *muscle memory*. It is akin to being able to turn off one's alarm clock without groping for it or, as will be discussed in later chapters, swinging the long cane exactly the same distance from side to side no matter what resistance in the terrain the cane tip encounters. An athlete learns to accomplish this kinesthetic movement when throwing a curveball or tossing a shotput. The best athletes learn to reproduce the closest-to-perfect motor skill under competition by visualizing themselves completing the necessary motor skills before they actually attempt to do so. This cognitive understanding facilitates the correct series of motor skills.

To reproduce these skills, one learns to control one's movements. Because motor strength and endurance dictate how well one can accomplish this task, students must be physically fit to be motorically efficient. Therefore, their physical conditioning should be assessed before instruction begins. Since many adults and children with visual impairments (especially elderly people and adults and children with additional impairments) lead sedentary lives, an assessment of their physical conditioning plays a vital role in the success or failure of any mobility program. A formal assessment should be conducted by a qualified physical therapist or an adaptive physical education instructor, who analyzes such factors as the integrity of the neuromuscular system, balance, coordination, body build, strength, cardiovascular endurance, muscular endurance, and flexibility.

The O&M specialist, classroom teacher, or rehabilitation teacher can conduct a functional assessment of a student's physical conditioning by observing the student performing motor tasks associated with game playing (rolling, kicking, tossing, and catching a ball), climbing a jungle gym, and doing jumping jacks and noting the student's posture and balance while standing, walking, and running and when performing various fine motor skills, such as pouring, sewing, knitting, and crocheting. Whatever the venue for observing skills, the assessor notes whether a motor skill is performed accurately and efficiently and later incorporates the results into a formal O&M program, in concert with the multidisciplinary team that is responsible for the student.

The following principles of learning must be kept in mind when developing a motor skills program:

1. An assessment must be done of what the student can accomplish both physically and cognitively.
2. The progression of stages of training is based on what the student can and cannot perform.
3. Positive, successful experiences must be provided in the early stages of learning.
4. Fear should be eliminated or reduced in the early stages of learning.
5. Overlearning motor skills should take precedence over rushing the student into the next stage of training.
6. The duration of practice sessions should increase after the student's level of skills increases.
7. Mental and verbal rehearsal of a skill speeds the acquisition and retention of the skill (Croce & Jacobson, 1986).

When a student is taught motor skills early in the mobility program (or in the student's life), the acquisition of later advanced motor and orientation skills will proceed more rapidly.

POSTURE AND GAIT

Maintaining proper postural readiness and efficient gait patterns goes hand in hand with coordinated motor skills. Persons with visual impairments often have poor posture because they may be insecure and afraid when moving about the immediate environment. In addition, without visual input, they have no point of visual fixation from which to judge verticality or uprightness. That is, without sight, one does not necessarily note that one is not looking up or straight ahead. As a result, many persons with visual impairments often exhibit one or more of the following postural difficulties: anterior head droop or tilt, rounded shoulders, dorsal kyphosis (a rounding of the upper portion of the back), scoliosis (a curvature of the spine), lumbar lordosis (an inward rounding of the lower back) with a protruding stomach, and pelvic tilt.

Compensating for Postural Irregularities

These postural abnormalities usually affect a person's gait patterns. For instance, to compensate for head droop, the person must counter the forward shifting of the center of gravity by widening the base of support, that is, by spreading the legs apart and toeing outward. To walk, the person will shuffle her feet while shifting or swaying from side to side. The overall effect appears to be a waddling forward. But to keep from falling to the side, the person will counterbalance herself by extending her arms out to the sides. Thus, overall she moves with what has been termed a "blind" gait.

A seemingly simple postural problem like head droop can cause a variety of other gait and conceptual problems. For example, by shifting the weight from side to side as she walks forward, the person will place more weight on one foot than on the other. This shifting from side to side can result in unintentional veering from the intended line of travel, which could pull the person into a parking lot or into the parallel street without her realizing it. When one's head is tilted downward, it is difficult to compensate for this problem by listening to and using the sounds of traffic to correct a veer because it is difficult to localize the sounds accurately. That is, one can confuse the sounds of traffic on one's side (the parallel traffic) with those of traffic on the perpendicular street.

Tilting the head, drooping the shoulder to one side, or toeing one foot outward all can affect the direction of the forward movement away from the intended line of travel. If these postural problems favor the right side of the body, the person will veer to the right. Thus, if the parallel street is on the person's right side and she veers to the right when attempting to cross a street, she will drift into that street and may step into moving traffic or onto the wrong street corner without realizing it. (For a detailed discussion of the ramifications of veering when crossing streets, see Chapter 8.)

Correcting Problems

The O&M instructor should correct the student's postural problems, if possible, before stressing efficient gait patterns and should do so in concert with a physical therapist because the instructor is not a licensed therapist. However, he can follow an appropriate behavioral management program with the guidance of the physical therapist (see Chapter 1). If it is determined that such a program will not correct the problem or problems, then adaptations to compensate for the deficiencies will have to be developed. For instance, with a student who veers to the right, the O&M instructor might teach the student to swing the long cane farther over to the left side of her body than would normally be expected to counterbalance the shifting to the right side.

As with proper posture, efficient gait patterns are normally learned through imitation. However, because a student with a visual impairment cannot see to imitate, she may require guidance and feedback on what it means to perform a motor skill properly. Therefore, the O&M instructor may need to place the student's feet in the proper heel, toe, and push-off positions through the gait sequence, show the student how to point her toes directly ahead or bend and hyperextend the knees to step down onto her foot or to push off the foot and onto the other foot, and show her how to swing her arms while walking forward.

Once these physical manipulations are introduced, they must be practiced during and between lessons to become ingrained. Parents, teachers, and rehabilitation professionals must all work together to reinforce these skills and behaviors. Without this unified effort throughout each day, the student is not likely to learn the skills and may not be able to use incoming sensory impressions to understand the world about her or may use them inefficiently.

SENSORY PERCEPTIONS: INTERPRETING ONE'S RELATIONSHIPS WITHIN THE ENVIRONMENT

The three main sensory perceptions that affect the orientation of a person with visual impairments are tactile, auditory, and visual. How well these perceptions are integrated into the person's repertoire of functional usage determines how well oriented she becomes in the environment. Although each type of perception is discussed separately here, all three must be integrated for the person to use the information efficiently to determine exactly where she is at a given time.

Tactile Discrimination: Elementary Perceptions

The first reliable and constant impressions of the world come to persons with visual impairments through the sense of touch. An infant grasps objects and brings them up to her mouth to taste, suck, and eventually chew on and further develops this sense by creeping and crawling about the crib and playpen. In the first year of life, a normally seeing infant comes to understand that if an object cannot be *seen*, it still may exist. The infant with a visual impairment learns the same principle of object constancy by coming to understand that even if she cannot touch something, it may still exist. Exactly how an infant develops this concept is unknown because the research on the impact of visual impairment on early cognitive development is limited (Scholl, 1986).

Over time, the child learns to compare, differentiate, and identify objects in the environment by the concepts of size, shape, weight, texture, temperature, and location. She learns that whether they are large or small, soft or hard, balls are still balls. She also learns that balls differ from bats, for example, by size, shape, weight, and texture and that balls can ricochet off bats, roll long distances, and bounce under other objects. These are invaluable concepts for understanding objects and interactions between or among objects in the environment, and they will be discussed in greater depth later in this chapter.

Auditory Discrimination and Localization: Intermediate Perceptions

If a person with a visual impairment were to rely solely upon tactile perceptions to understand the environment, the breadth and scope of her knowledge would be limited. Therefore, she needs to learn to discriminate and localize the myriad sounds around her to extend her knowledge away from her body. These ambient sounds are either informational or extraneous. By knowing exactly what to listen for (and what to weed out) and when to use such sounds, the person with a visual impairment greatly enhances her ability to maintain her orientation.

DISCRIMINATING SOUNDS

To discriminate or differentiate among sounds effectively, one must be exposed to and be given feedback about different sounds and sources of sounds. Usually, these sounds are paired with their sources by being touched or seen. For instance, as the infant with a visual impairment flails her hands about, her hands inadvertently touch the mobile overhanging her crib, which emits a sound (a melody or jingling of bells, for example). Over time, she learns to associate the sound with the object. If she hears the sound in the future, she recognizes that it comes from the mobile and reaches up purposefully to find it.

As the infant grows into a toddler and then into a young child, she associates more and more objects that emit sounds with their sounds, and vice versa. As the environment becomes more familiar to her, she begins to look for associations among objects and the sounds they emit. Later, in the mobility program these sounds take on even more significance in determining positional relationships. For example, the sounds of constant typing emanating from the principal's office indicate a potential landmark to the young schoolchild with a visual impairment. If she becomes disoriented while walking in the school's halls, she can listen for the sounds of typing and walk toward them, locate the office door, and then reorient herself to get back on track to reach her intended destination. Likewise, many children and adults are able to differentiate among sounds so well that they can identify individuals simply by listening to their footsteps.

LOCALIZING SOUNDS

Localizing sounds is a more difficult task than simply discriminating among them. Because sounds have unique characteristics, they are affected by a number of variables. The pitch, tone, medium, and direction of sounds can be confused by the distance from the source of the sounds, the environmental conditions in which they are heard, and the presence of competing or extraneous sounds. Sounds can be muffled or appear to be distant on snowy days as a result of the direction of the wind and whether a traveler is wearing a hood, cap, or face mask to shield herself from the elements. They can appear to be closer and louder on rainy days. They can be masked or muffled by the droning of louder, competing sounds. And they can be shadowed or muted by objects between their source and the individual. Thus, a person may think traffic sounds are a half block away when they are really several blocks away, simply because the wind is blowing toward her from the sources of the sounds. On snowy days, the traveler may not hear an oncoming vehicle until it is right next to her because the snow beneath the tires muffles the sounds on the pavement. And a pedestrian in any large city may confuse the direction of traffic sounds because of the echoes created by the tall buildings.

SOUND-LOCALIZATION ACTIVITIES

A person who is visually impaired must be given enough real experiences in a variety of environmental situations to learn to make accommodations to these unusual conditions. But first, she can learn to localize sounds through a variety of exercises. The O&M instructor can present his voice and have the student follow it in an open gymnasium or auditorium and, eventually, throughout the hallways in a school or agency. Over time, the student learns to keep the instructor's voice in front of, alongside of, or directly behind her.

The instructor can use other sources of sound, such as clickers, bells, metronomes, and audiotapes of music and traffic, to achieve the same objectives. He mixes movements, walking alongside the student while the student is stationary, having the student move while he himself remains stationary, and having both of them move. He varies the distances of the sounds from being close to the student to being much farther away.

Later, these skills become important when the student attempts to walk parallel to traffic without walking into the street or into a parking lot. If she veers into the parking lot or any other wide open space, she can use the parallel cars along her side or the perpendicular cars, which are directly in front of or behind her, to leave the area.

As the student becomes more proficient in using localized sounds, she learns to create her own sounds to understand better the positional relationships among objects in the space around her and herself. This learned ability used to be thought of as the sixth sense of blind people. Later it was called "facial vision." Today it is called *echolocation*. For instance, as the student approaches a wall directly in front of her, she learns to note the echoes emanating from the wall that are created by her footsteps or by other contrived sounds, i.e., by snapping her fingers, lightly clapping her hands, or making clicking sounds with her mouth. The farther away from the wall she is, the greater the echo; the closer she is, the shorter (if any) the echo. It is best to learn to use this skill by using natural and available sounds to create the echoes and not to call attention to oneself in a socially inappropriate manner.

By learning to develop this skill, the traveler further refines the quality and efficiency of her travel abilities. She does not have to bump into the wall in her path to recognize where it is located. She can hear the intersecting hallway on her side as she enters it without having to trail the wall surface. She can differentiate among open and closed doors along a wall to her side. And she can walk into a room and snap her fingers to each side of, in front of, and behind her to determine by the echoes (or lack of echoes) the approximate size and shape of the room and whether she is next to one side wall or another.

Relying solely on sounds to understand one's location in the environment is problematic because sounds are affected by so many variables. By pairing sounds with available tactile evidence and information, however, one can make reasonable deductions about true positional relationships. For example, by listening to the sounds of the typewriter in the principal's office and finding an available wall, the student can determine which hallway she is in, her position, and which direction she is facing in relation to those sounds.

Visual Discrimination: Advanced Perceptions

Vision is the most extended of the distance senses we humans have; we can see farther than we can hear or touch. If a person's vision is limited in acuity or field of view, her mobility will be either significantly or tangentially affected. The definition of *legal blindness* is a central visual acuity of 20/200 or less in the better eye with correction, or a central visual acuity of more than 20/200 if there is a visual field defect in which the peripheral field subtends an angular distance no greater than 20 degrees in the better eye. People with an acuity of 20/200 can see at 20 feet what those with "normal" vision can see at 200 feet. A person who has the use of only one eye would not be considered legally blind if her visual acuity was greater than 20/200 or if she had a peripheral field wider than 20 degrees (National Society to Prevent Blindness, 1980). Although the range of types of low vision could be from normal acuities with restricted fields to light or object perception only, it must be noted that the vast majority of individuals with visual impairments have some degree of usable vision.

Assessing Functional Vision: Practical Approaches for the O&M Instructor

It is imperative, therefore, that a low vision specialist (optometrist or ophthalmologist) first determine what a person with a visual impairment is seeing or not seeing and under what conditions (her visual efficiency). No two people with the same visual acuity or visual fields will make use of their visual experiences in the same ways. And on any given day, one's vision may fluctuate—from what one has seen previously or even a few minutes before an assessment. The multidisciplinary team of professionals involved in the person's case uses the assessment of visual efficiency to develop a program to help the person use her remaining vision better. If the team concludes, after consulting with the low vision specialist, that low vision aids may be useful in this process, such devices will be introduced into the training program, as appropriate. These aids may include monocular telescopes for distance viewing, hand-held magnifiers for near viewing for short periods, and closed-circuit television (CCTV) magnification systems for longer reading periods.

Low vision assessments can be either formal or informal. Both types of assessments should be performed for each individual. Formal assessments are conducted by the low vision specialist in a clinical setting. The specialist determines a person's visual acuity and fields of view at near and distant ranges, the proper lighting conditions to read text, and any low vision aids that may aid near and distance viewing.

Informal, or functional, assessments are done by an education or rehabilitation professional in the actual environmental settings, to determine the visual skills necessary to complete a particular task or tasks. The education or rehabilitation teacher is concerned with the person's ability to identify objects in the immediate environment, to scan along a page of text visually, to identify shapes and colors, and so forth. The O&M instructor is concerned with the person's ability to locate and identify objects in both the immediate and remote environments. However, all the professionals wish to learn similar things about the student's or client's visual fixating, scanning, and tracking of objects, both stationary and moving. They may go about their assessments in different ways to reach similar conclusions. The focus of this discussion is on the O&M instructor's assessments.

VISUAL FIXATION

The O&M instructor wishes to determine how quickly and easily the student can visually locate and focus on an object or target (also called *visual fixation*). By having the student look at targets or objects at various distances away and then point to them, the instructor ascertains vital information about the student's fixating abilities. By having the student do this exercise in different settings and under different lighting conditions, the instructor begins to piece together a picture of the student's overall visual fixating abilities.

IDENTIFYING OBJECTS

After the student can detect some object in her field of view, she must then identify that object in some manner—on the basis of the object's size, shape, color, or location or some previous visual memory of it. In any event, it is important to avoid erroneous conclusions based on initial impressions. For instance, if the assessment is conducted in a location that is known to the student, familiarity may bias the results. It is best, therefore, to conduct all or part of the assessment in an unfamiliar environment.

While the instructor walks with the student along a hallway, for example, the instructor can ask the student to identify objects along the walls or on the floor. Asking effective questions without giving answers is an important part of this process. For instance, the instructor may ask the student to locate an object halfway down the hallway and along the right wall and to point to it. If the student does so, the instructor may then ask her to try to identify the object. The student may say it looks like a table. If the instructor answers yes (or no), he has reinforced the student's reliance on him for instant identification of the object. However, since he wants to know exactly at what distance the student can truly and confidently identify objects, he needs to resist the temptation to give an answer and ask the student to walk toward the object and to stop when she can truly identify it without guessing. He then notes the distance and lighting conditions. He can estimate the distance either discretely (10.5 feet away) or less discretely (about one-third of the way down the hall). He determines the lighting conditions by using a light meter or, more functionally, by noting that the hallway is dimly lighted, well lighted, or brightly lighted. He will continue this task in various indoor and outdoor settings.

VISUAL SCANNING AND TRACKING ASSESSMENTS

Another way to assess visual functioning is to ask the student to walk various indoor routes to locate numerous objects. For instance, the instructor may ask the student to go from the rest room on one floor of a building to the soda machine on another floor without being told exactly where the soda machine is located. As the student walks the route and explores the new floor, the instructor monitors how the student handles the exercise visually by observing her from all sides. That is, does the student visually scan (or move her eyes back and forth to find stationary objects) both sides of the hallway? How well does she visually track moving objects and identify room numbers? Does she grope with her feet at the stairwells? Does she look down at her feet when walking? Does she stop and let her eyes readjust (or accommodate) to a change in lighting conditions, or does she just continue walking? And, does she bump into objects as she moves along? A similar exercise can be conducted outdoors in a parking lot or a street, where the student can be asked to identify street names and addresses; signs; and various visual landmarks, such as light poles, parking meters, benches at bus stops, and fire hydrants. By observing the student's behavior in a variety of settings and lighting conditions, the instructor can put more of the pieces of the visual functioning puzzle into place.

Visual tracking assessments can also be performed indoors or outdoors. For example, the student can be asked to track moving objects (passersby in hallways and on streets and traffic outdoors) visually and to point at these moving objects as they pass across or along her visual field. If the student loses track of the moving targets, she may have some problem with her visual fields.

ASSESSING VISUAL FIELDS

One way to assess the student's *nasal* (closest to the nose) and *temporal* (off to the sides) visual fields is by asking her to sit in a large auditorium or gymnasium and to keep one eye closed while fixating the other on a target directly in front of her. The instructor walks into the student's visual field from various distances from the right side and then from the left side and asks the student to tell him when he has done so and places an object on the floor in that location. The instructor then repeats the exercise by starting within the field of view and walking out of it. He assesses the student's visual field in the other eye by repeating both exercises. The various objects in front of the student at the end of this assessment represent the boundaries of the student's visual fields in functional terms.

The instructor next checks the student's *superior* (upper) and *inferior* (lower) fields by having her fixate on his face close up while he moves a penlight or other object in and out of the respective fields. He also asks the student to follow overhead lights in a hallway by keeping them centered just above her head or to one side as she walks along or outdoors and to walk along sidewalks with overhanging awnings, tree branches, and so on or with lamps and other objects protruding from buildings. In addition, he asks the student to identify descending stairs or curbs at a distance and then walk up to them and stop—or does not let her know they are there and determines if she detects them visually as she approaches them (ensuring her safety if she does not detect them). By comparing these results with the information on the nasal-temporal fields, the instructor has vital information on the student's current functional use of her visual fields.

The assessment of how well a student is using her remaining vision will be used to determine how extensive a low vision O&M program should be developed. Formal fixating exercises may be devised, along with scanning and tracking exercises. The assessment activities just described can become formalized training exercises.

Eventually, the student must be able to use her vision efficiently to walk safely through the environment while visually noting where she is and what she is passing or coming upon along the way. How well she is able to do so will determine which low vision aids, if any, will be required to assist her in this process.

NONOPTICAL LOW VISION AIDS

Nonoptical low vision aids are objects or devices that do not require a prescription by a low vision specialist. For O&M instruction, these aids may include sunglasses or caps with visors to reduce glare, felt-tip marking pens used with contrasting colored paper to make low vision maps, reading lamps and stands, and painted strips or textures in contrasting colors that are placed on landings and stair steps. These aids are usually simple answers to particular low vision problems.

OPTICAL LOW VISION AIDS

Sometimes a low vision problem is complex enough to require an aid, such as eyeglasses, a prism to expand visual fields, a monocular telescope to view distant objects, or a magnifier to view small print, that must be prescribed by a low vision specialist. Although some aids may be purchased directly from a camera shop or stationery store, they should still be prescribed by the low vision specialist. For instance, the instructor may believe that a hand-held magnifier will solve a student's immediate problem reading the prices on canned goods, but if he prescribes the aid, he may not detect an underlying visual problem. Therefore, the instructor should refer the student to an optometrist or ophthalmologist for an eye examination and share his ideas with the low vision specialist. The specialist will then check for underlying physiological problems and allow the instructor to try out a particular aid.

VISION SIMULATION DEVICES

In the course of the low vision assessment or training program, the O&M instructor evaluates the student's abilities to function visually. Over time, he may determine that the student is receiving too much extraneous visual input. That is, the student seems to be confused about what information she is receiving, to the point where she literally closes her eyes to shut out the input. In such a case, the instructor must decide what approach to use to help the student distinguish between information that is usable and information that is not. Some instructors prefer to use blindfolds or occluders and to instruct their students as if they were totally blind. However, it takes only a little experience with this approach to discover that students will revert back to using (or being confused by) their vision once the occluders are taken off. Thus, it is not advisable during instruction to simulate total blindness or to prepare students for the possibility of total blindness. Rather, students must be taught to use whatever remaining vision they have more efficiently, even if their visual prognosis is poor.

Some low vision simulators simulate various visual acuities, say, of 20/70, 20/100, 20/200, 20/400, and 20/1000. Others simulate field restrictions that are typical of certain eye conditions. These conditions are characterized by a blurring of the entire field (cataracts or high myopia), a blurring or total loss of the central field (macular degeneration), a blurring or total loss of the peripheral field (retinitis pigmentosa), or a total loss of various halves (hemianopsias) or quarters (quadrant anopsias) of the fields of view. These aids are generally used to demonstrate a student's field restrictions to interested persons in the community and to the student's family members. They should be used judiciously because they do not truly simulate the eye conditions and could lead some to make erroneous comparisons or conclusions about the visual functioning of their friends or loved ones.

TEACHING CONSIDERATIONS FOR LOW VISION STUDENTS

How well a student uses her remaining vision depends on a number of factors. Some of these factors are directly related to the student's visual problem, whereas others are related to the visual circumstances; the student's age; the student's educational and cultural backgrounds; and any other physical, emotional, and cognitive difficulties. The process is further complicated by the encouragement and support of those who have a significant impact on the student's life.

The low vision curriculum must be incorporated, then, into the entire O&M program. It cannot simply be used after certain isolated skills are taught, but must be presented in conjunction with the teaching of those skills, whether they be long cane skills to detect objects below the waist and drop-offs at curbs and stairs or the ability to locate addresses and street signs while walking along a sidewalk. For all the reasons mentioned, the O&M curriculum for many low vision students may be much longer than the curriculum for students who are totally blind. Throughout the text and at the end of each chapter, additional teaching considerations for individuals with low vision are presented.

CONCEPT DEVELOPMENT AND ENVIRONMENTAL AWARENESS

People who are blind or visually impaired may not understand positional relationships between themselves and objects in the environment. How do they relate to objects they cannot see? Where are these objects in relation to them? What happens if they move away from objects: Are the objects still behind them or off to one side?

These and other concerns have important implications for students' ability to remain oriented. Without a firm understanding of spatial and environmental concepts, their mobility will, indeed, be limited.

Understanding Spatial and Environmental Concepts

Concepts are concrete, functional, or abstract mental representations, images, or ideas of what something should be. *Concrete concepts* can be identified by specific characteristics. For example, a baseball may have a round shape, a smooth surface, a leathery skin, and stitched seams and be too hard to squeeze. Functionally, it is hit, tossed, thrown, and caught in a game. To have an abstract concept of a baseball, one would have to be able to recognize it by seeing it, touching it, smelling the leather, and hearing a bat striking it or a glove catching it and somehow recall those characteristics to develop a mental representation of what it looks, feels, smells, and sounds like and what one could do with it.

Concept development is the process by which people learn to understand the various characteristics of objects and their relationships to one another and to themselves in the environment. How well they learn these characteristics depends, in great part, on how well they integrate the incoming sensory perceptions to form a holistic view of objects and space about them. Because concept development depends mainly on visual input, people who are blind or visually impaired have greater difficulty understanding concepts in their abstract forms. Thus, although models, maps, and pictures help people gain a better understanding of the characteristics of such objects as the moon, sun, and stars, without the aid of the visual sense, it is difficult to understand the depth and scope of the galaxy, the universe, and the vast distance among and between stars and planets. Simple representations of such vast positional relationships do not readily show the magnitude of the distances between them as well as do telescopes or pictures taken from observatories or satellites. However, one who has a visual impairment can still develop a personal definition and consistent understanding of such concepts, even in abstract terms. The following discussion of the relationships of various types of concepts to the acquisition of O&M skills is based on Hill and Blasch (1980).

Spatial Concepts

The knowledge of objects in space and their relationships to each other is essential to maintain or regain one's orientation. After a person with a visual impairment understands her body and body parts by developing a sound body image, she is then better prepared to explore the objects in the space around her. These objects can be in front of or behind her or above, below, under, next to, beside, far from, close to, inside or outside, opposite, parallel, or perpendicular to her. Other spatial concepts describe spatial relationships associated with cardinal compass directions (north, south, east, west, southwest, northeast, and so forth) or with the position of objects to the Earth (diagonal, horizontal, and vertical).

Still other concepts relate to the shape and form of objects—such as circle, square, triangle, rectangle, sphere, and cylinder—and letters are used to describe the shapes of street patterns or hallway configurations—T-intersection, H-hallway, and Z-route. In addition, some concepts involve measurement: inch or foot; minute or second; ounce or quart; wide, narrow, thick, or thin; mile; less, more, all, or none; tall, short, or long; and big, tiny, and great.

As a person develops an understanding of these positional concepts, she naturally compares them to herself: Is the object larger or shorter, above or below, next to or far from me? This self-to-object comparison is critical to the understanding of positional relationships. She then compares an object to other objects. Object-to-object comparisons include similar questions. Individuals with visual impairments derive answers to these questions by walking over to and exploring the objects, but always first asking, How does this object compare to me in distance, size, and shape?

Functional Assessments of Spatial Concepts

O&M instructors must learn exactly which concepts their students truly understand and which their students confuse or completely misunderstand by assessing their students' attainment of concepts using the proper assessment instruments. A number of such instruments are available: the Body Image of Blind Children (Cratty & Sams, 1968), for children aged 5-12; the Orientation and Mobility Scale for Young Blind Children—Short Form (Lord, 1969-70), for children aged 3-12; the Stanford Multi-Modality Imagery Test (Dauterman, 1972), for children aged 16 and over; and the Hill Performance Test of Selected Positional Concepts (Hill, 1981), for children aged 6-10. For a brief comparison of these instruments, see Hill (1986) and Hill and Blasch (1980). Some instruments are reliable and have proven validity, while others do not. How the instrument is to be used will determine which tool is correct for assessing a child's concept development. At the time of this writing, there are no reliable or valid instruments to test the spatial concepts of adults with visual impairments. However, one can assess an adult's spatial awareness and understanding informally while asking her, for example, to walk along a hallway on the right side, locate the third door from the end of the hall, and use her upper forearm while protecting herself.

In any event, the student should be allowed to demonstrate her understanding of the aforementioned terms of positional relationships in a variety of ways, either formally or informally. The instructor can devise a checklist of terms and can ask the child to manipulate a few tools in a variety of ways. He can observe the child playing such games as Simon Says, Treasure Hunt, Follow the Leader, and Red Light/Green Light or ask the child to place objects under, over, and within one another or to position herself beside, between, next to, above, or under some objects. As the child or adult learns certain mobility skills, she can be asked or reminded to use her right hand, stay parallel with the right side of the hallway, hold on to the guide's left elbow when walking with a sighted guide, and so on.

Environmental Concepts

To move through the environment effectively and efficiently while maintaining one's orientation throughout, one must understand the objects one is most likely to encounter along the way. Environmental concepts can be recognized according to their shape, temperature, texture, and location (Hill & Blasch, 1980). Among the numerous concepts related to travel are these: city, residential, business, traffic light, traffic, cars, buses, trains, planes, taxicabs, city blocks, neighborhood, road, street, parkway, tree lawn, intersection, grid pattern, cul de sac, traffic circle, offset intersection, T-intersection, traffic lanes (live and dead), shoreline, grassline, lawn (yard), bush, flower, weed, landmark, path, fence, house, wheelchair ramp, curb cut, ceiling, floor, hallway, room, stairs, landing, parking lot, light switch, and elevator.

CUES AND CLUES

As a traveler walks through an environment, she must ascertain which objects will be helpful in maintaining her orientation and which should be ignored at a given moment. Some concepts are cues and others are clues. *Cues* are critical objects or the sounds emitted from those objects that trigger instant recognition of one's location. For example, hearing someone use the only water fountain on a floor may tell a student that she is in the same hallway as her classroom and that she is trailing along the same side of the hall as the classroom. *Clues* are secondary objects or sounds emitted by those objects that help one piece together one's exact location. A student may not yet know her exact location upon identifying the clue, but by pairing it with other pieces of information or other clues, she can eventually determine her exact location. For example, since there are several water fountains on a particular floor, the student cannot determine her exact location from hearing one being used. But she can explore farther along a hallway wall to locate some other object, such as another classroom or office, to determine that she is in the desired hallway and traveling in the intended direction. Clues, then, can lead to cues.

CONCEPTS OF TEMPERATURE

As was mentioned earlier, some concepts can be used according to characteristics other than their location in space. Concepts of temperature are important for planning travel. Knowing that it is hot and muggy out may warn the traveler to plan to travel earlier or later in the day. If it is cold and icy, she may plan her route to walk along the sunny side of the street or to start in the afternoon when the ice has had a chance to melt. Some important temperature concepts related to mobility are hot, cold, warm, cool, mild, chilly, icy, muggy, windchill, humid, dry, centigrade, and Fahrenheit.

CONCEPTS OF TEXTURE

Textures of terrain are also important concepts to understand. Whether walking paths are rough or smooth, soft or hard, jagged or bumpy, or wet or dry will affect one's travel plans. Travel surfaces have various textures that will affect the type of cane skills the traveler uses. Some of these surfaces are pavement, cement, asphalt, stone, macadam, gravel, dirt, and mud and may be leaf-, snow-, or ice covered.

CONCEPTS OF TIME

Concepts of time play an integral part in one's ability to understand the environment. Some of these concepts are second, minute, hour, day, week, month, year, today, tomorrow, yesterday, half hour, quarter hour, morning, afternoon, evening, and night. As the person with a visual impairment gains proficiency in travel skills, she will begin to plan out her routes to meet certain schedule requirements. She will learn to plan enough time for emergencies that may arise, such as having to walk alternate routes to avoid construction sites or making sure that she has enough time if she becomes disoriented along the way.

CARDINAL DIRECTIONS

Finally, the traveler must make use of cardinal directions if she is to be truly independent in her travels. It is not enough to know lateral directions of right and left, for if she were to turn along the route, objects that were once along her right or left side may now be in front of or behind her. Cardinal directions enable her to take into account objects on all sides of her in a constant and consistent way. They can be true, relative, or contrived. True cardinal compass directions relate to north, south, east, and west. They can be related to the position of specific, touchable objects in the immediate environment, such as the north wall of a room, or of more distant objects, such as north of the river. They can be related more discretely to the environment, for example, the northeast corner of the intersection or the southwest corner of the floor, or can be relative to the environment in that travel can proceed in a northerly direction if the street and sidewalk do not run true north-south. No matter how the traveler turns as she moves through space, the cardinal directions remain fixed; only her relationship to the directions changes. However, when the traveler does not know any of the true compass directions in a specific situation, she can then use contrived compass directions. For instance, if she walks into an unfamiliar building without first noting the directions, she can simply decide that "north" will be in front of her as she enters the building. As long as she keeps the directions consistent from that point onward, she can still maintain her orientation using compass directions. Once she learns the true directions, she can reorient herself accordingly.

Linear Concepts

Individuals with visual impairments must learn to walk in straight lines to understand the true relationships of objects in the space about them. The understanding of linear concepts is integral to self-sufficient mobility. But one must first understand the concept of a "point" before one can understand the concept of a "line." Points can be found in everyday life in such things as buttons on a shirt or on an elevator. They can be the place on which one stands (one's point of origin or reference point), on every step one takes, and where one eventually winds up (one's destination point). They can be represented by staccatolike sounds, as in the rat-a-tat of a jackhammer or the backfiring of an engine. By using a multisensory approach to learning, then, the instructor helps the student integrate the concept into a truer comprehension of the term.

Lines are an accumulation of points. They can be arranged in a row to form a straight line or about an arc to form a curved line. For persons with visual impairments, straight lines provide a greater understanding of positional relationships, especially the concept of opposites. What is opposite the entry door in a room? If I locate the bulletin board in the hallway, will I find the drinking fountain opposite it on the other side of the hall? And how will I know I have reached the opposite corner on the other side of the street? These are just some examples of questions about the environment to which the traveler with a visual impairment must find answers. Without the concept of opposites, her ability to solve these situational problems will be severely limited.

One type of straight line may be perplexing to the student, however, when she is trying to define or describe certain positional relationships: a diagonal line that moves across two different planes simultaneously, frontally and laterally. For example, that the northeast corner of an intersection is actually the southwest corner of the block, or diagonally opposite, or that the window in a particular room is diagonally opposite the reference door, may be especially confusing. For the student to understand this relationship, she must use herself as the reference point, be able to point to objects in front of her, and be able to walk from one object to another directly opposite. Therefore, the concept of diagonal must succeed the understanding of straight ahead of or directly opposite oneself. (For a more detailed discussion of the importance of the relationship among objects in a room, see room-familiarization procedures in Chapter 5.)

Furthermore, straight lines can be combined at one or more points to form different configurations. These configurations help the traveler better visualize the shape of the route, where she is on the route at a particular time, and where she needs to go to complete the route to reach her destination. These route shapes can be described and demonstrated using the English or braille alphabet. The four basic route shapes, using the English alphabet, are the I, L, U, and Z (or stair-step) shapes and their reversals. All route configurations are merely derived from these shapes. And when the traveler with a visual impairment combines these configurations with other information (compass directions, names of streets or hallways, and landmarks along the route), she is well equipped to maintain her orientation or to regain it if she becomes disoriented. The understanding and use of route shapes are predicates for successful mobility skills. (For a more detailed discussion of this concept, see Chapter 4.)

When teaching concepts to children or adults who have visual impairments, the O&M instructor must take into consideration the age and cognitive levels of the students because children and adults can be shown certain concepts and experience them in the environment in different ways. Children benefit from playing games like Simon Says, Red Light/Green Light, and Mother, May I? They can learn their body parts and how to move through space properly by imitating others in their play activities. They can learn concepts like straight and diagonal by playing beep baseball or goalball. They can learn about up, over, under, and around by playing on jungle gyms, swings, or trampolines.

Adults, on the other hand, need to learn or relearn concepts in more indirect ways that do not demean them as individuals. They can learn about parallel and perpendicular by walking along a wall in a hallway or by listening to traffic sounds as they walk on a sidewalk. They can be constantly reminded of their left and right sides as they hold a sighted guide's arm or when they grasp a cane and swing it from side to side. For adults, concepts should be integrated directly into the curriculum without calling attention to them.

Whichever concepts are determined to be deficient must be attended to if the individual is to understand the space around her and to maintain her orientation. Without this knowledge and understanding, the traveler with a visual impairment may not travel the road to independence efficiently.

3

Basic Techniques
for Guiding a Person
with a Visual Impairment

The four basic methods of travel for persons with visual impairments are the use of the sighted guide technique, the long cane, the dog guide, and electronic travel aids. The sighted guide technique is the primary travel method in which persons with a visual impairment use the assistance of someone who has vision. Essentially, in this technique, the person with a visual impairment holds on to the sighted person's arm in a particular fashion while the two walk along together. Because it is usually the topic of the first formal lesson in the traditional O&M curriculum, the basic sighted guide technique provides students with the first opportunity to exercise some control over the environment. The student has the right to accept or refuse the assistance. And even after he has accepted help, he can reject it at any time simply by letting go of the guide's arm.

In working through the curriculum, the instructor precedes each O&M skill with an explanation of the reasons for using the skill and for performing it in a specific manner. With all the skills, the instructor encourages the student to question why he is being asked to do things in a particular manner; if the answers are unsatisfactory, the student should not be required to do them. As the lessons and units progress, the instructor listens carefully to the student's concerns and relates, when appropriate, her training, experiences, and frustrations in similar circumstances as a means of helping the student know that she can empathize and sympathize with his predicament.

All O&M lessons are sequenced so that one skill is learned before the next is taught. Each technique may be thought of as a mini-unit with several lessons devoted to teaching and practicing the skill, if necessary. Therefore, the basic sighted guide skill may be taught over several lessons until both the instructor and student seem confident that the skill has been learned.

The instructor carefully selects environments suitable for lessons. Indoor areas that are quiet, relatively free of pedestrian traffic at first, and have progressively more complex areas to traverse are ideal for initial sighted guide lessons. For instance, for teaching and practicing basic sighted guide skills, an area should have long corridors with intersecting hallways. Later lessons in the unit would incorporate travel areas with hallway "furniture," such as chairs, benches or couches, drinking fountains, coat racks, and stairs, that allow the instructor and student to practice traveling through narrow passageways and doors and on stairs. Areas that develop from light to moderate to heavy pedestrian traffic are necessary as well.

The sighted guide procedures lay the foundation for building a trusting relationship and a positive rapport between the instructor and student. The student begins to learn that the environment can be negotiated safely and with confidence. Although the environment may seem confusing at first, the instructor shows the student that there is, indeed, some order to this confusion. Stairs, elevators, rest rooms, and drinking fountains, for example, usually are located in the same relative locations on each floor in a particular building, and the numbering systems in a particular building are likely to be consistent from floor to floor as well. The student, who begins the O&M program with numerous preconceptions, apprehensions, and travel experiences (both positive and negative), must learn to trust that his instructor will not let any harm come to him during the course of instruction. Therefore, it is imperative that the instructor be knowledgeable about her student's background, health concerns, and motivation to learn O&M skills to pair lessons with the student's travel goals. The successful matching of the student's goals to the lessons will enhance the mobility program and ensure positive professional relationships between the partners. Upon completing the sighted guide procedures, the two should be able to walk as a team through any travel environment and situation with confidence and safety, and the student should be able to teach these procedures to future sighted guides.

PROCEDURES AND PRINCIPLES
Basic Sighted Guide Procedures

- The prospective guide (hereafter referred to as the instructor) offers assistance to guide the person with a visual impairment (hereafter called the student). Usually, the offer is made verbally, as in, "Would you like to take my arm?" or "Would you like to go sighted guide?" The student may initiate assistance by asking, "May I take your elbow, please?" or "Let's walk together sighted guide." The instructor uses a calm, reassuring voice and gives the student positive, verbal feedback when the student performs the skills satisfactorily. Many persons prefer to walk holding onto a certain arm of a sighted person simply because they prefer to use the dominant hand or because one hand is weaker or has less feeling than the other. The instructor defers to the wishes of the student at first, but will show him that there are many situations in which it is preferable to use the other arm when walking through a particular travel area.
- If the offer is accepted, the instructor extends one arm toward the student and lightly touches his arm so there is no need to grope to find the extended arm.

- The student grasps the instructor's closest arm slightly above the elbow with his thumb along one side and his fingers wrapped around the other side (see Figure 3.1A). The grasp should neither be too tight nor too loose: it should be comfortable for both persons yet secure enough for both to feel each other's movements and responses to environmental situations as they walk together, such as approaching stairs and obstacles in their path.
- The student stands alongside, facing the same direction, and approximately one-half step behind the instructor with their shoulders almost touching. This position is extremely important because it allows the instructor to monitor the student when they are both maneuvering through potential obstacles and barriers in the environment. The student becomes an extension of the instructor's arm.
- As the instructor walks, the student maintains the same body and spatial positions (see Figure 3.1B). The two remain alongside each other, almost shoulder to shoulder and within a half step of each other, even when the pace varies or when they gradually turn in either direction. Moreover, when they walk down a different corridor or turn to walk in the opposite direction, the instructor or student can be the pivot point about which the other turns, depending on the direction or necessity of the turn.
- The grasp is usually broken by mutual agreement. It is courteous for an instructor to explain to the student where they are standing when she stops guiding him. If a student is to be left alone, the instructor guides him to a stationary object like a chair, table, or wall, rather than leave him in an open space where he may have difficulty determining his location and exact orientation to the room.
- If the student wishes to release his grasp of the instructor's arm, he simply lets go.

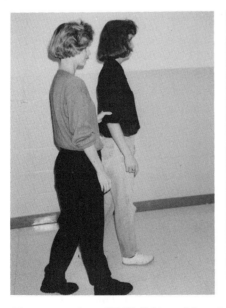 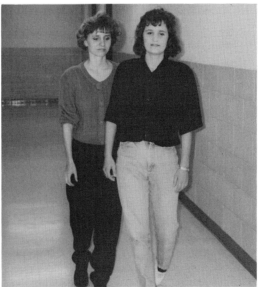

Figures 3.1 A and B Walking with a sighted guide: The basic sighted guide position.

Special Situations and Variations

In everyday life, people who are blind or visually impaired encounter a wide variety of situations that require variations on the sighted guide technique. Descriptions of these variations as performed by instructor and student follow.

REVERSING DIRECTIONS: ABOUT FACE

It may be necessary in some situations for the instructor and student to turn around and stand or walk in the opposite direction, yet there may not be enough room to negotiate the turn by pivoting in a congested area, such as a crowded hallway or an elevator. Therefore, the turn may be facilitated by using the about-face procedure.

• The two reverse their direction by executing two 90-degree turns. First, they turn 90 degrees to face each other while the student continues to grasp the instructor's guide arm.

• The student then grasps the instructor's free arm slightly above the elbow, which is extended out toward him, so he can find it.

• The student lets go of the original guiding arm after grasping the free arm, and the two then complete the procedure by executing the second 90-degree turn to face in the opposite direction (see Figures 3.2-3.5).

TRANSFERRING SIDES

As they walk together, it may be necessary for the instructor to ask the student to walk holding on to the instructor's other arm to avoid barriers or hazards along the route or simply for convenience. The procedure for transferring sides is as follows:

• While in the basic sighted guide position and still grasping the instructor's arm, the student steps behind the instructor and grasps the instructor's guiding arm with his free hand, so both hands are now grasping the instructor's same arm, slightly above the elbow.

• The student then lightly runs the back of the hand that originally had grasped the instructor (with the fingers relaxed and slightly cupped) along the instructor's

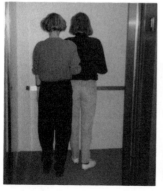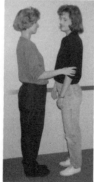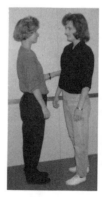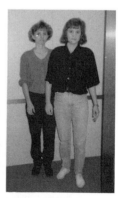

Figures 3.2-3.5 Reversing directions while entering an elevator: The about-face technique.

back until he finds the instructor's free arm. The student then grasps the free arm just above the elbow and releases his grasp of the original arm.

- As the student crosses behind the instructor, and with the newly freed hand, he grasps the new guiding arm so that both hands are now holding this arm just above the elbow. He then frees the first hand that had grasped this arm and assumes the proper sighted guide position on the side opposite the side on which he was originally positioned.

This procedure should be practiced several times while stationary before the two attempt to accomplish it while walking. The instructor can assist the student by extending her free arm back slightly while the student is beginning the transfer to avoid confusion in locating the arm. While walking, the two can facilitate the transfer and prevent the student from tripping over the instructor's heels by slowing down their pace, by the instructor's shortening her stride, and by the student's extending his arms almost to arm's length during the transfer.

NEGOTIATING NARROW PASSAGEWAYS

Often, the instructor and student cannot travel together in the basic sighted guide position because the travel environment has narrowed as a result of obstacles and barriers along one side or the other. In such a case, the narrow-passageways procedure should be used:

- The instructor positions her guiding arm behind and across her back, bent at the elbow and out away from the body.
- The student, while maintaining the grasp of the sighted guide technique (slightly above the elbow), steps directly behind the instructor and at arm's length, to avoid tripping over the instructor's heels. Without turning at the torso, the instructor periodically looks over the shoulder of her guide arm to monitor that the student is, indeed, directly behind her. The arm of the hand the student is using to hold on to the instructor is diagonally across his body. The two slow down their pace and shorten the length of their strides.
- After the narrow area has been traversed, the instructor will reposition her guide arm back alongside her body, and the student will return to the normal sighted guide position.

The instructor has the option, especially at first, to tell the student when to go into the narrow-passageways position. However, after the two have traveled together for some time, it should not be necessary to verbalize the need because the change in arm position should be enough to indicate that the student should implement the procedure. As they practice together, the two use this procedure to walk through all narrow spaces, including open doorways (see Figures 3.6-3.7).

NEGOTIATING CLOSED DOORS AS A TEAM

After some time working together, it will be necessary for the instructor and student to go through doors that are closed. Since the two are acting as a team, each has specific responsibilities when negotiating closed doors: the instructor opens the door and the student closes it behind them after they have passed through it. The

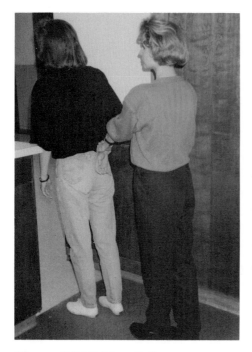 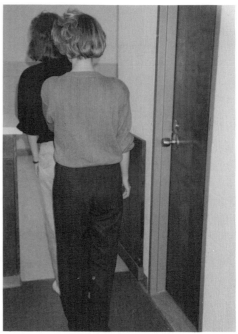

Figures 3.6-3.7 Negotiating a narrow space with a sighted guide.

instructor walks directly up to the closed doorknob or push bar to within a few inches, or "kissing distance," of the door. The instructor explains to the student that doors normally open four ways: toward them, away from them, to their right side, or to their left side. Doors are opened using two of these four ways. That is, they will open toward you and to your right, away from you and to your left, and so forth.

It is important not to confuse the student with erroneous (confusing which side or which way) or ambiguous information (the door jam is on the left). At first, the instructor tells the student the lateral direction of the door opening and whether it is opening toward or away from them. In the correct position, the instructor begins to open the door and simultaneously exaggerates a turn at her torso in the direction of the door opening. Eventually, this overturning will cue (or signal) the student to the direction in which the door has been opened without having to verbalize the information. That is, if the student feels the instructor moving forward and turning in toward him, he will learn to interpret this cue as the door opening toward them and to the same side as he is positioned. After the two begin working as a team, it will no longer be necessary to verbalize the information; they will be able to carry on incidental discussions without interrupting them with directions on what is happening along their route.

The sequence is developmental, from the simplest situation to the most difficult. In the first situation, the door opens toward the instructor and student and to the side on which the student is standing (the easiest situation to learn in that it does not necessitate a repositioning of the student, and the body cues are the easiest to discern):

- As the instructor opens the door with the hand of her nonguiding arm (as will always be the case), she exaggerates the turning movement toward the student, and the two step backward several steps to feel the direction of the door opening (in this case, in toward them). Some instructors believe that their students should never have to back up and will stand far enough away from the door so that when it swings toward them, they are able to stand still.
- The instructor opens the door only as far as her guiding arm's shoulder.
- The student places his free arm across his body at shoulder height for protection from the oncoming door edge and places his hand on the edge of the instructor's same shoulder to find and hold on to the door edge. Thus, the student knows exactly where the door will always be positioned and will not have to grope for it (and potentially miss it, which could cause injury).
- The student accepts the door edge from the instructor and extends the door open, so the instructor walks through the doorway first and the student follows while still holding on to the door with one hand and the instructor with the other.
- After they have gone through the doorway, the student slides his hand down to the doorknob, holds on to the knob, and closes the door behind them. He then lets go of the door and reassumes the sighted guide position. If the door automatically swings shut, he simply lets go of the door after they have cleared the doorway area (see Figure 3.8).

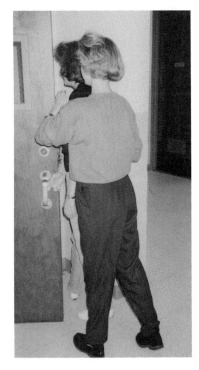

In the second situation, the door opens away from the instructor and student and to the side on which the student is standing:

- The instructor walks to within kissing distance of the door to reinforce the body movements without the need for verbal feedback later, explains how the door will open, opens the door and exaggerates the turning movement toward the student, and begins to walk forward. The door is opened only as far as the instructor's shoulder once again, so the student will know where to find the door without groping for it.
- The student positions his free arm across his body for protection so that his hand touches the instructor's shoulder.
- He then accepts the door from the instructor and opens it completely so the two can walk through the doorway.

Figure 3.8 Negotiating a closed door that opens toward the team.

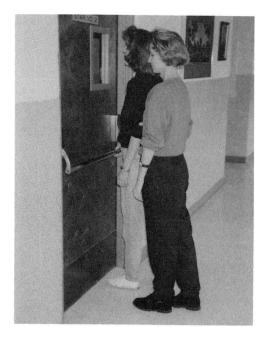 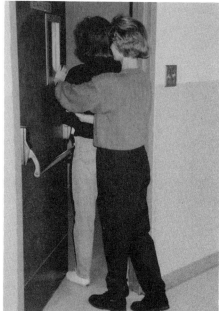

Figures 3.9-3.10 Negotiating a closed door that opens away from the team.

- After both have passed through the doorway, the student closes the door behind them (see Figure 3.9-3.10).

In the third situation, the door opens toward the instructor and student but to the side on which the instructor is standing:

- The instructor, within kissing distance of the door, explains how the door will open, begins opening the door, and backs up slightly while turning her torso away from the student.
- To grab hold of the door while maintaining contact with the instructor, the student executes a new procedure, the partial switch: He grasps the instructor's guiding arm with his free arm and then steps behind the instructor at arm's length; he frees the original arm and places it across his chest for self-protection in finding the door edge. He then completes the procedure as follows:
- The student glides this hand along the instructor's back until he finds the back of the instructor's shoulder opposite the original guiding arm's shoulder.
- Meanwhile, the instructor opens the door only to this shoulder, so the student can easily find the door edge.
- The student grasps the door edge and opens the door far enough so the two can walk through the doorway together.
- Once they have passed through the doorway, the student releases the door or closes it behind them and reassumes the original sighted guide position.

In the fourth situation, the door opens away from the instructor and student and to the side on which the instructor is standing:

- Within kissing distance of the door and after explaining how the door will open, the instructor begins opening the door and steps forward while turning away from the student; she opens the door only enough for her to walk through.
- The student effects the partial switch and reaches out for the partially opened door.
- The instructor looks to see how far to open or close the door so the student can find it, and once the student has a hold of it, she lets go.
- The student grabs hold of the door and walks through it with the instructor and then closes it behind them and assumes the original sighted guide position (see Figures 3.11-3.13).

NEGOTIATING STAIRS AS A TEAM

It is important for the student to begin to rely on the instructor for information about the environment and for safety; this is the primary reason for teaching procedures for negotiating stairs without using handrails first. The instructor explains the procedure in its entirety before beginning it. The two will first practice ascending stairs because it is less threatening to most students than is descending stairs.

The procedure for *ascending stairs* is as follows:
- The two approach the ascending stairs squarely so that the instructor's toes are touching the first riser and the student is about a half step behind in the basic sighted guide position.
- The instructor begins the ascent first; the student follows so that he is one stair step behind the instructor. (For balance and safety, the instructor may hold on to the handrail on the side opposite that of the student.)
- When the student first steps onto the landing, the instructor gently pulls the guide arm (and the student) forward to indicate that there are no more stair steps on that particular flight of steps. The two then move quickly and carefully away

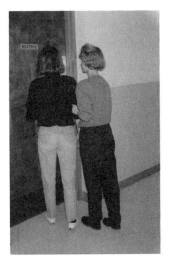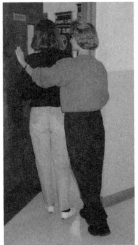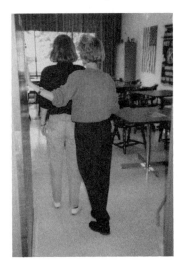

Figures 3.11-3.13 The partial switch while going through a closed door.

from the edge of the landing and are ready to attempt the next flight of steps in the same manner. It may be necessary to give some students a verbal cue or simply to pause as they step onto the landing. For other students, it may be more appropriate to teach this procedure first using handrails, especially if the students are fearful on stairs or have balance and coordination problems.

It is best to begin at the bottom of several flights of steps to practice the procedure without having to negotiate descending stairs. As the two negotiate the stairs, the instructor observes the student to ensure balance and safety and establishes a rhythm of stepping onto one step above the student at the same time the student steps onto the step below. Later, the student also seeks to establish that rhythm so that both traverse stairs in tandem. The student leans forward slightly throughout the ascent to maintain his balance and a forward momentum. Both should avoid stopping on any step during the ascent, and each should place one foot on each step throughout, rather than place two feet on a single step.

To *descend stairs*, the following procedure is used:

- Before the descent, the instructor guides the student to a wall at the top of the landing that is directly opposite the stairs to discuss the procedure, so they do not totter at the edge of the stairs. With the student's back to the wall and the instructor standing in front of and facing the student, the instructor explains the stair-descending procedure in detail.
- While using the sighted guide technique, the two approach the descending stairs perpendicularly (directly facing) and stop at the top of the stairs with the instructor's toes over the edge of the step; the student is a half step behind. The instructor monitors the student's position to ensure that he is in the "ready to descend" position—squarely facing the steps with his head, shoulders, hips, and toes pointing directly ahead.
- The instructor begins the descent, and the student follows so he is one stair step behind the instructor.
- When the student places his foot on the landing at the bottom of the stairs, the instructor gently pulls the guide arm forward to pull him forward, as was done during the stair-ascension procedure. The two walk over to the next flight of stairs and practice the procedure accordingly.

It is best to begin at the top of several flights of steps to practice the procedure without having to negotiate ascending stairs. As the two negotiate the stairs, the instructor once again observes the student to ensure his balance and safety and establishes a rhythm of stepping onto a step at the same time the student steps onto a step. Later, the student also seeks to establish that rhythm so that both traverse stairs in tandem. The student leans backward slightly throughout the descent to maintain his balance. Both should avoid stopping on any step during the descent, and each should place one foot on each step throughout, rather than place two feet on a single step. The instructor may need to remind the student to bend at the knees during the descent, especially if the student shows any signs of anxiety (such as rigidity).

After teaching the procedures for both ascending and descending stairs, the instructor introduces the student to using the handrail, as follows:

• The instructor guides the student to the stairs and with her free hand places the student's free hand on the handrail.

• As they negotiate the stairs, the student glides his hand along the handrail and slightly ahead of his body while maintaining the sighted guide position.

• When he feels the end of the handrail, he lets go of it. The instructor points out to him, however, that stair railings can begin after the first stair step, can end prematurely, can wind around a staircase, or can be nonexistent. Therefore, it is preferable to rely upon the sighted guide for stair negotiations whenever feasible.

In some circumstances, however, it may be preferable for the student always to use the handrails when negotiating stairs. Students who have conditions associated with age or being overweight; hearing disorders; or diseases, such as multiple sclerosis or muscular dystrophy, may need to use the handrails for precautionary measures, as well as for balance and support.

FINDING AND SITTING IN A SEAT

Proper seating procedures are one form of refinement that help the student develop confidence in travel, especially when other people are present. Specific procedures can be used for sitting down gracefully and safely in various situations.

For *sitting in a free-standing chair*, this procedure is used:

• The instructor approaches the chair squarely, so the student's knees gently make contact with the front of the chair.

• The instructor explains how the chair is positioned relative to the student and places the student's hand that is on the guide arm on the back of the chair.

• The student takes his free arm and places it across his body and in front of his face for protection and then bends slightly forward at the knees and allows the free arm to find the chair seat.

• The student explores the chair seat for objects that may have been left in it, and if none is present, grasps the arms of the chair, turns around, and sits down. He learns to follow this procedure quickly and gracefully, practicing it with various chairs.

For *sitting on a couch or sofa*, the same procedure is used:

• For courtesy, the instructor informs the student exactly where along the couch he is seated, that is, at one end or in the middle of the couch. She also informs him whether and where others are seated on the couch.

For *sitting in a chair at a table*, the following procedure is used:

• The instructor guides the student to the chair so the student's body gently contacts the back of the chair and explains their position relative to the chair and table.

• The instructor places the student's hands on the back of the chair and then guides the back of one hand to locate the table's edge. The back of the student's hand is used because it is possible to miss the edge and knock over some object on the table with his fingers.

- The student, maintaining one hand on the back of the chair and the other on the table's edge, moves to the side of the chair and pulls it out from under the table.
- He then checks the chair seat for objects with the hand that had been pulling the chair out from the table.
- If no objects are found, the student, maintaining his hand and body weight on the table rather than on the chair, sits in the chair and pulls himself up to the table's edge without letting go of the table edge with the one hand, if possible. If he places his weight on the chair when sitting down, he quickly learns that a chair is less stable than a table and may have casters that can cause it to roll out from under him (see Figures 3.14-3.18).

ACCEPTING OR REFUSING ASSISTANCE: THE HINES BREAK

The Hines break is the first of several role-playing procedures in preparation for the student's eventual daily meetings with the public, including family and friends. This procedure, named for the Veterans Administration (U.S. Department of Veterans Affairs) Hospital in Hines, Illinois, where it was developed, enables the student to determine how he will be guided or whom he will or will not allow to be his guide in temporary circumstances. It should be reinforced and practiced throughout the remainder of the O&M program:

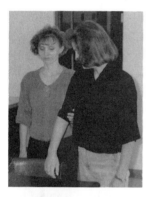
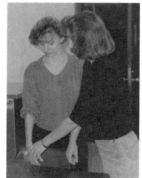
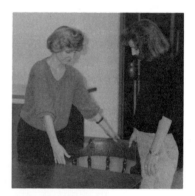

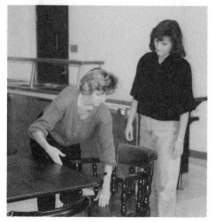
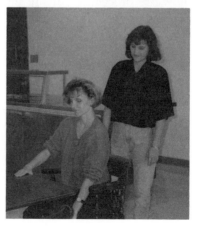

Figures 3.14-3.18 Taking a seat in a chair at a table.

- The student stands in an open space with both arms at his sides.
- The instructor approaches the student from behind and to one side and verbally offers assistance to him while grasping his arm above the elbow (and begins pushing the student forward).
- If the student wishes to accept the offer but to have the individual assume the proper sighted guide position, he pulls the arm being grasped across the front of his chest to break the grasp.
- At the same time, he takes his free hand and grasps the instructor's wrist from underneath their arms by wrapping his fingers and thumb around the instructor's wrist from its underside (for better leverage) and pulls the wrist downward to break the grasp entirely.
- While holding onto the instructor's wrist, the student slides his freed hand to just above the elbow of the instructor's arm and assumes the proper sighted guide grasp and position.
- As an alternate method, the student can make his arm limp when it is grasped, rather than bring it across his body. Doing so makes it extremely difficult for someone to drag him along until he initiates the correct grasp (see Figures 3.19-3.23).

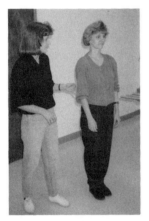
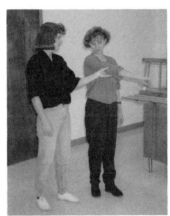
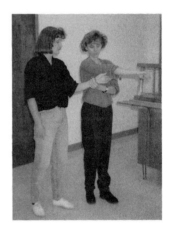
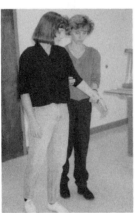
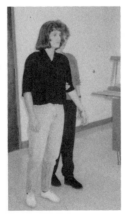

Figures 3.19-3.23 The Hines break.

While using either procedure, the student politely thanks the instructor and tells her that he would rather take (or hold on to) her arm. If the student wishes to reject the offer of assistance entirely, he simply lets go of the instructor's arm after breaking the hold and politely refuses the assistance.

This procedure should be practiced numerous times with either arm being suddenly grasped until the student feels satisfied with the procedure and reacts quickly to each role-playing situation. The instructor should "surprise" the student periodically throughout the O&M program so the response becomes automatic and appropriate. The student learns that the public can offer assistance at the least-expected times, so he must be prepared to react without thinking; otherwise he may be escorted across a street he has no intention of crossing.

The student responds in a firm but polite manner because most people are well intentioned but often uninformed about how to approach a person with a visual impairment. The student may be the first person with a visual impairment that a sighted individual encounters and, as such, has a responsibility to educate that person in a positive manner.

GUIDING TWO OR MORE PERSONS AT ONE TIME

If the instructor has to guide more than one person at a time, she does so in a chainlike manner. That is, the second person to be guided holds on to the student's free arm in the proper sighted guide position, the next person holds on to the second individual's free arm, and so on. The obvious drawback to this procedure is the amount of space taken up by the chain, but the positive aspect is that each person in the chain can perform all the other sighted guide skills without having to modify them. Although other procedures are possible and acceptable, the instructor should take into account the travel environment and the level of skills of those she is guiding.

GUIDING PERSONS IN AUDITORIUMS AND SIMILAR AREAS

People who are blind or visually impaired need to use certain techniques to negotiate rows of seats in such areas as auditoriums and theaters. The instructor can teach these techniques in the following way:

• The instructor enters the row first, facing forward, and the student, using the basic sighted guide grasp of the instructor's arm, follows, sidestepping along until the instructor stops with the student directly in front of the vacant seat. The student may run his free hand along the back of the seats in front of him as he sidesteps into the row, as long as he is careful not to make contact with persons sitting in those seats.

• When exiting the row in the same direction as they entered, the instructor arises first and steps in front of the student and across to his other side. The student then rises and grasps the instructor's arm in the sighted guide technique, and they exit sidestepping out of the row accordingly. It is important for the instructor to enter and exit the row first. It is courteous for the instructor to inform the student of their relative position in the auditorium once they are seated. That is, the student should be told the location of the stage, the loudspeakers, the exit doors, and the approximate row and aisle positions. This information can be critical in emergency situations when the two may be separated.

GUIDING PERSONS IN CAFETERIAS

Cafeteria lines present another special situation that calls for specific techniques. There are two possible procedures to follow when the instructor and student practice negotiating cafeterias together:

• The instructor may guide the student through the cafeteria line using one tray for them both (or for the student first and later for herself), pointing out the various food items and prices, placing the items on the tray, and guiding the student through the line to pay for the meal and on to the table.

• If the two have separate trays, the student sidesteps along the cafeteria line following the instructor by scooting his tray alongside her tray. After paying, the student lifts the tray with one hand draped over the far side of the tray, which is propped up against his waist and above the belt, while the other hand is braced under the tray for stability. The student follows the instructor either along one side while touching the instructor's arm or shoulder with his arm or shoulder or behind the instructor, lightly touching the instructor's back with the tray. Although it is recommended that the instructor carry all glasses, cups, and other liquid containers to avoid possible spills as they make their way to the table, this precaution is not always necessary. Many people prefer to carry their own items on their own trays. If the student is carrying a long cane, he can slip it under the arm he is using to brace the tray and hold it across the body diagonally to act as a bumper to locate tables, chairs, and other obstacles in the path (see Figures 3.24-3.26).

CONSIDERATIONS FOR EFFECTIVE TEACHING

Paying attention to certain refinements can maximize the effectiveness of instruction. Consideration of fine points and individual needs is a vital part of teaching and reaching the student.

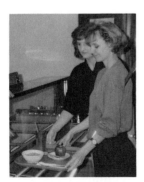 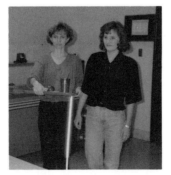 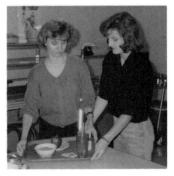

Figures 3.24-3.26 Guiding through a cafeteria line and finding a seat.

Guiding the Student

As they walk together, the instructor should use the guiding arm to keep the student close by, tensing it slightly and bringing it closer to the body in tight situations or relaxing it and moving it slightly out from the body under normal conditions. The instructor's guiding arm can be held relaxed at her side when she is walking or slightly bent at the elbow, either pointing directly in front of her or across her body at waist height. The pace should be slow at first but pick up over time until both instructor and student feel comfortable. Walking too slowly causes both of them to wobble and bump shoulders; walking too quickly will cause the instructor to drag the student.

Developing a Kinesthetic Feeling for the Skill

For the student to learn what the guided arm position should feel like, the instructor can place the student's arm in the correct position and then do the following isometric exercise: After the arm is positioned, the student relaxes his grasp and lets go of the instructor's arm. Facing the student, the instructor then holds on to his hand and arm (halfway between the wrist and elbow) and asks him to press the arm forward and tense it while maintaining the position, and then to relax it while maintaining the position. The instructor asks the student to repeat this procedure several times, and they then practice the correct sighted guide procedure.

Modifying the Grasp

The basic grasp of the instructor's arm can be modified to fit the student's age, height, or other physical characteristics. Small children or shorter persons may have to grasp the arm farther down from the elbow or on the wrist. Preschoolers may grasp one or two fingers. Likewise, taller individuals may have to grasp the arm higher up than just above the elbow. Persons with balance problems can grasp the instructor's arm, which is bent at the elbow and extends directly out from and in front of the body, between the elbow and the wrist with one or both hands and with the fingers and thumbs wrapped around the arm for added leverage. If two hands are used, the hand closest to the instructor wraps around the instructor's arm from underneath and then over, and the other hand is placed on top of the instructor's same arm. Care should be taken not to hold on to the instructor's shoulder because one cannot receive proper body cues in this manner.

Under certain circumstances—generally when lighting conditions are poor or there is a lot of glare—students with low vision may need to rely on sighted assistance temporarily. It may not be necessary to expect them to use every sighted guide procedure or to demonstrate the same level of efficiency as do their counterparts who are blind. On the other hand, some students have little usable vision and must rely on a sighted guide more often. Whatever the expectations, however, low vision students must know when, where, and under which conditions they are to use sighted assistance.

Using Landmarks, Cues, and Clues

As the lessons progress, the instructor can incorporate the rudiments of orientation into the instruction. The student explores landmarks, which are objects or a configuration of objects that are fixed, identifiable (visually, auditorially, or tactilely), and unique to an area. Indoor landmarks include elevators, drinking fountains, rest rooms, bulletin boards, soda and candy machines, and stairwells. The location and relationships of common objects are critical for using them as landmarks. For example, there may be several drinking fountains on one flooor of a building, but only one may be located next to a particular secretary's office. Some environmental objects or situations, such as the sound of a typewriter or other equipment in the secretary's office or of someone drinking from a water fountain, may cue the student as to his current location. Environmental cues signal in the student's mind an instant recognition of his location.

Clues, on the other hand, provide information that the student must decipher to lead to a proper (or improper) deduction as to his relative location in the environment. Clues are generally added to other pieces of information to arrive at a general conclusion. For example, when a student estimates the distance traveled down a hallway to be about halfway and feels a sudden change in the temperature of the air along his side of the hallway, coupled with the sound of a typewriter, he may conclude that he is next to the secretary's office. The instructor begins to include these pieces of information about the travel environment in the lessons because they will become more important to the student in future lessons.

Knowing When to Move On

The sighted guide skills should be reinforced throughout the O&M curriculum each time the instructor and student walk together to, during, and from lessons. Therefore, it is not imperative for students to learn each aspect of the sighted guide technique perfectly before moving on to the next procedure. Instructors will know that it is appropriate to move on to the next skill when their students relax their grasps, consistently demonstrate proper positioning and reactions to the instructor's body and verbal cues, and have been given various opportunities to demonstrate the transfer of skills to different travel environments. Students generally exhibit a tight grasp at first, but as they become familiar with the technique and begin to trust their instructors, their grasps become looser and more relaxed. Thus, the tightness or looseness of a student's grasp is one way to monitor understanding of, comfort with, and use of this skill. Instruction, therefore, should be reinforced on various floors of the same building, in different buildings, and even outdoors. Culminating lessons to the unit should include practicing all skills in various travel environments, which should make the lessons both practical and more interesting for both students and their instructors.

Teaching Others the Sighted Guide Skills

By the end of the sighted guide unit, the student learns how to teach the sighted guide procedures to both strangers who will temporarily guide him through travel environments and to relatives, friends, and associates who will be acting as guides over longer periods. The student needs to teach only those skills for which the guide must take the responsibility, that is, those that require the guide to inform him of upcoming situations. The student knows what to do in those instances and does not have to tell the guide all the details, for example, that he will be stepping behind her and grabbing the door with his free hand.

On rare occasions, students may need to guide other blind persons. These situations may arise at an agency or school for blind people or when the student is traveling indoors with a friend who has a visual impairment. To role-play such a situation, the instructor should act like the other person with a visual impairment, respond as if she is unfamiliar with the technique, and follow the student's commands literally. She should not blindfold herself or impair her vision in any semipermanent manner because she must monitor and provide instant feedback for the student's lead in critical situations (as they cross open corridors or pass by doorways or near stairs, for instance). It is during these culminating lessons that students learn how to take control over their environment and truly begin to travel on the road to independence.

4

Self-Protection Techniques: Moving through the Environment Independently

After students learn the sighted guide techniques, they may have gained enough confidence and feel more ready to move through the environment with another person. Other skills may now be introduced to build upon this foundation to enable them to move through the environment independently. Using the procedures described throughout this chapter, instructors can teach their students the basic self-protection techniques for avoiding protruding and oncoming objects and for trailing or gliding the hand along a wall's surface to ensure safe travel.

THE TEACHING ENVIRONMENT

The instructor structures the lessons to consider the teaching environment, the developmental sequence of the lessons, and the routes used for practice and reinforcement. The same environment used for sighted guide techniques will also be conducive for teaching self-protection skills. Lessons once again progress developmentally; skills are introduced separately and then combined to form another skill. For instance, before learning to trail a wall, the student learns to use the upper hand and forearm self-protection technique because it is required for trailing along a wall while walking.

Some skills are performed to avoid or anticipate problems. For example, when the student turns right to walk down an intersecting hallway, she uses her left upper hand and forearm as she walks out in open spaces. If she cuts her turn too sharply, she risks running into the corner of the two hallways. Therefore, she will learn to contact the corner with her hand, rather than her elbow (as she might have done had she used her right arm in the upper hand and forearm position), since she is less likely to injure herself using her hand. The instructor constructs lessons that allow the student to practice traveling in various situations, such as walking into open spaces and then trailing specific walls to locate a door to a room, trailing a wall to another objective and then walking into open spaces to complete the route, and estimating distances down a hallway and then trailing a wall to the destination. All these situations are practical and are predicates for upcoming lessons on using the long cane both indoors and outdoors.

In addition to reinforcing the learned skills, these lessons help the student become familiar with the indoor environment. Even though formal techniques for familiarizing oneself to various indoor and outdoor environments are not usually taught at this stage, the very nature of the teaching process helps the student learn the environment. By mixing travel situations with protection skills, the instructor should be able to develop 15–25 separate routes locating various destinations in just one hallway.

This chapter, then, outlines the sequential process that is used to help ensure that one skill is built on another. When walking without a long cane or other travel aid, the student uses the learned skills only in familiar, indoor environments because they provide little to no protection from overhanging objects, objects contacted below the knees, or stairs.

SELF-PROTECTION TECHNIQUES

When not using a sighted guide, people who are blind or visually impaired often use skills related to the upper hand and forearm technique, the alternate hand and lower forearm technique, and trailing to move safely through the environment.

Upper Hand and Forearm Technique

- With her back to a wall or closed door at the end of a long corridor and with the instructor in front of and facing her, the student touches her opposite shoulder with the back of her hand.
- She then extends her hand from her shoulder and out in front of her to arm's length. The instructor ensures that the hand is in front of the opposite shoulder, palm out, and that the arm is parallel to the ground and extended but not locked at the elbow. The fingers are slightly cupped, and the hand is relaxed. In this position, the elbow can receive objects as glancing blows that will not cause injury to it or to the upper arm. The shoulder is relaxed and can be massaged by the instructor if tight, and the other arm is relaxed at the student's side.
- An alternate method is for the student to place her arm directly out in front of her chest and bent at the elbow, so the forearm is parallel to the ground and forms a 90-degree angle at the elbow, the palm faces away from the body, the fingers are slightly cupped, and the hand is extended slightly past the opposite shoulder.

The Alternate Hand and Lower Forearm Technique

While using the upper hand and forearm technique, the student learns to place the alternate hand and lower forearm across the groin area, with the arm extended slightly from the body and the palm facing the body. The arm and hand are relaxed, and the fingers are slightly cupped. This technique protects the student from some objects below the waist, such as chairs and tables. The skill can be used without the upper hand and forearm technique in indoor areas with which the student is familiar. The skill is learned using either arm and hand in position.

Monitoring the Student's Progress

When the student first walks out into open spaces, the instructor uses the "follow my voice" technique to ensure the student's safety and straight-line travel and to reduce the student's anxiety. In a hallway, for example, the instructor faces the student and asks her to follow his voice down the hallway. As the student walks along the corridor, the instructor periodically says, "Follow my voice," and offers such words of encouragement as, "You're doing great; keep coming at me"; "You're looking fine; keep it up"; "terrific"; and "super" (see Figure 4.1).

The instructor also provides verbal feedback to the student on how well she is performing the technique and where she is in the hallway. For instance, as the student walks down the hallway in open space using the upper hand and forearm technique, the instructor may say, "You're doing great, but please rotate your palm outward more," or "Raise your arm a little higher." The instructor does not tell the student that she has veered to her right, which can be confusing when she is concentrating on moving her upper hand more to the right. Rather, he moves closer to the student and asks her to come toward his voice, which forces her to pay more attention to her location in the environment but does not cause her to confuse the laterality of her hand position with that of her body position. As the student gains experience and is able to accomplish the objectives of a lesson, the instructor lessens the frequency of his verbal comments until he no longer provides them.

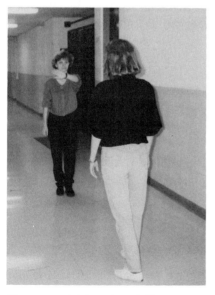

Figure 4.1 Using the "follow my voice" technique during a lesson on the upper forearm procedure.

The instructor on occasion presents a barrier to the student when the latter walks in an open space by placing his arm in front of the student as she approaches. This action shows the student that the upper hand and forearm technique does, in fact, detect obstacles without causing injury to the face. It is done in a nonthreatening manner and only when the student becomes adept at using the technique. As the student progresses to the point at which the instructor no longer thinks it is necessary to stand or walk in front of her, the instructor follows behind or walks alongside the student. He looks for various aspects of the technique to provide appropriate feedback. From behind, he should be able to see the upper hand just beyond the student's opposite shoulder, and from the side, he should be able to see the full arm extension. As the student walks down a hallway, the instructor can stand halfway down the hall and watch her from all three positions: the front, the side, and behind as she walks by.

THE FIVE-POINT TRAVEL SYSTEM AND ROUTE PATTERNS

As the lessons progress, the student learns that she must integrate and make use of additional information when traveling to maintain her orientation throughout the environment. The instructor begins to show her what to attend to when walking and gradually introduces her to the *five-point travel system*: the route pattern or shape, the compass directions, the names of the hallways (and later of streets), the landmarks along the route, and all the above in their reverse order on the return trip.

To move from one location to another, the student walks in one of four basic route patterns or shapes, or its derivative. The basic patterns, in order of their complexity from simple to difficult, are expressed using letters of the English alphabet: I, L, U, and Z (or stair step). The instructor can draw these patterns on the student's palm or back, depending upon the preferred visualization plane. If drawn on the palm, the letters are traced from the base of the palm toward the fingers, or from the body forward and in the direction of the initial phase of the route; if drawn on the back, the instructor traces the letters from the lower back to the upper back. In either case, the patterns will appear to be upside down to the print reader. That is, to trace an L–shaped route on the back, the instructor starts at the lower right-hand side (or left-hand side, depending upon the direction of the next phase of the route) and traces a straight line up to the upper right-hand side (just below the right shoulder blade) and straight across to the upper left-hand side (just below the left shoulder blade). The letter is traced in this manner to illustrate the exact direction of the route. (If the student were to bend over at the waist so her back was facing the ceiling, the route pattern would be traced the way it was traced in her palm.)

If the student is a braille reader, these patterns can be expressed using configurations involving the braille cell: the I–route may be formed by connecting dots 6, 5, and 4; the L–route is formed by connecting dots 6, 5, and 4, and then dots 4–1; the U–route connects dots 6–4, 4–1, and then dots 1, 2, and 3; and the Z–route connects dot 6 to 5, 5–2, and then 2–1, as illustrated in Figure 4.2. A pegboard with rubber bands connecting the various configurations of pegs is an excellent aid for learning the concept of route patterns.

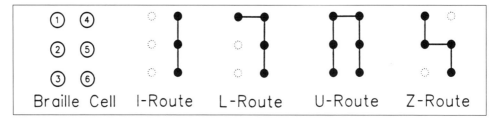

Figure 4.2 The braille cell used to illustrate the four basic route shapes.

As the student learns the route patterns, the instructor includes cardinal compass directions along with the route shapes. For instance, while facing north, the student walks an I–route from the south end of the corridor to the wall at the north end; while facing north, the student walks an L–route, north and then west; while facing north, the student walks a U–route, north, west, and south; and while facing north, the student walks a Z–route, north, west, and north. The student learns that an I–route requires no turns and that at the destination she is facing the same compass direction from which she started the route. Likewise, an L–route requires one lateral turn so that she ends up facing 90 degrees to the right or left of the original compass direction. The student further learns that both U– and Z– routes require two lateral turns but that she faces the opposite compass direction after completing the former and faces the same compass direction after completing the latter; yet, she will be in two different locations on the floor! For many students, compass directions can be introduced earlier in the program while teaching sighted guide skills. Examples of route patterns incorporating compass directions are presented in Figure 4.3.

To accomplish a turn on a route, the student will need to become aware of and use certain landmarks, which must be identified by their locations in particular hallways. Therefore, the hallways are designated by a distinguishing landmark (hallway names are replaced by street names later in the program). For instance, one hallway may be named the elevator hallway, and another, the rest-room hallway, if both are unique to that floor. For the Z–route, for example, the student walks north down the elevator hallway along the west wall until she comes into contact with the fifth door; she then turns east and crosses the hall and turns back north and trails along the east wall of the elevator hall until she locates the north wall of the rest-room hallway. To return to home base, the student must imagine the shape of the route, the compass directions, and the halls and landmarks in their reverse order and then complete the route accordingly.

The instructor provides the student with numerous opportunities to travel various routes and their reversals. He should expect, however, that the student's self-protection skills will suffer somewhat as she concentrates on her orientation skills, because motor skills are temporarily in conflict with cognitive skills until the former become nearly second nature to the student. This phenomenon will occur at the beginning of every unit of instruction in which motor skills are emphasized and

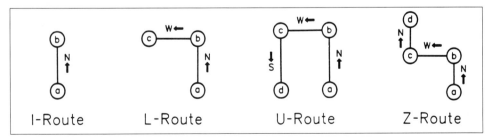

Figure 4.3 The braille cell used to illustrate route patterns and compass directions.

should dissipate by the end of each unit. The instructor's awareness of it should lessen his concern about the effectiveness of his teaching and reduce his initial expectations for the student.

The five-point travel system is integrated into every lesson in some manner from this time forward, so the student learns exactly what to be thinking about when she is walking. The student begins to realize that by keeping these five points in mind, she will find it increasingly more difficult to become disoriented or confused about her location in the travel environment.

TRAILING A WALL

After having walked in open spaces isolating the uses of the upper hand and forearm and the alternate hand and lower forearm techniques, the student now learns to trail along a wall. This technique is useful for maintaining one's direction and for locating objects or destinations found along the wall line, such as doors, elevators, drinking fountains, and bulletin boards.

- The student stands beside and parallel to a wall, with the wall along one side and with her shoulder almost brushing up against the wall. She extends her trailing arm (the one closest to the wall) forward to arm's length, waist high with the palm flat against and touching the wall. The fingers are then cupped so the fingernail of the pinky is all that is lightly touching the wall as the hand glides along.
- She places the opposite arm in the upper hand and forearm position, with the hand nearly touching the wall. This position will enable her to locate any objects projecting from the wall at head height, doors suddenly opening out into the hallway, or people unexpectedly walking out from offices. The student maintains these positions while walking forward.
- As an alternate trailing hand position, the student places the edge of the entire pinky finger against the wall.
- As a second alternate trailing hand position, the student places the back of the hand against the wall as it lightly glides along the surface.
- In a third alternate position, the student walks along the wall, brushing the knuckle of the first finger against it, the other fingers of that hand cupped together.

Although the alternate positions may feel and look more natural than the standard position, they can cause injuries. The skin can be scraped and bruised as the hand glides along the wall, especially on rough surfaces like brick and concrete; the fingers can be caught on doors and other objects; and for persons with diabetes who may have poor circulation or neuropathy in their hands, these injuries could develop into sores and ulcers (which, if not attended to, could ultimately involve possible risk of amputation of a finger). The standard technique, however, will provide every student with feedback in the proximal portion of the extremity, or the shoulder, which is generally unaffected by poor circulation and is, therefore, better able than are the hands to discern positional variations. If she strays from the wall, the student will feel a slight muscle strain in the shoulder of her trailing arm, which should consistently indicate the need to change her position.

As the student walks along when trailing, the instructor stands in front of, beside, or behind her, providing feedback about the correct positioning. If she does not maintain the correct position, the instructor adjusts the hand and arm placements as she moves along the wall line to reinforce the correct, rather than the incorrect, position while in motion. The instructor monitors the student to ensure that her head, shoulders, and feet are all in alignment while walking. The shoulder of the trailing arm should be relaxed while trailing. If it is tense, the instructor can massage it while the student moves along the wall.

Drifting away from the wall is natural at first and can be caused by the head or feet being turned away from the wall or by the body generally drifting away from the wall. If the student's head is turned away from the wall, the instructor asks her to "look at" the wall when walking. If the student's body drifts away from the wall, the instructor stands beside the student and lets her bump into him until she learns the correct position without bumping into the instructor.

The student practices trailing along one side before practicing trailing along the other side of her body. Therefore, the instructor takes her back to the starting point each time while using the sighted guide technique. After the student separately trails along either side, the instructor asks the student to practice going back and forth along the wall line in either direction without being guided to one end or the other. He allows the student to experience locating various objects along the wall that can be detected using self-protection techniques while protecting the student from objects above the chest and below the knees that cannot be so detected.

Crossing Open Doorways while Trailing a Wall

After the student has practiced trailing along a wall with no openings, she learns to cross open doorways (see Figures 4.4-4.5):

• The student trails along with one arm and uses her upper hand and forearm technique with the other arm. As she locates the near-side door jamb with her trailing

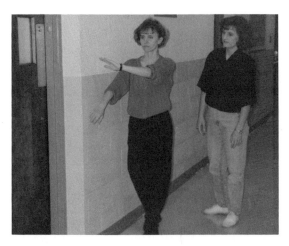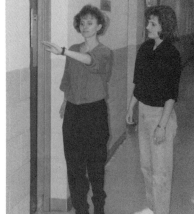

Figures 4.4-4.5 Trailing a wall and crossing over a doorway.

hand, she grasps the jamb and walks forward parallel to the opening until her upper hand and forearm locate the jamb on the opposite side of the opening.
• She releases the near jamb and then the second one after resuming trailing with the original trailing hand.

This procedure ensures that the student will not inadvertently walk out into an open space and lose her intended line of direction and travel. If the opening were to a corridor, for example, the student would not have lost hold of the wall when reaching for the opposite side. She would still be able to stay with the wall and analyze the situation to determine which path to follow, using one of the procedures described next.

Squaring Off and Aligning

The student is ready to learn to negotiate open corridors after having practiced walking across open doorways because corridors are generally wider crossings than are doorways. There are two ways to cross wide open areas while maintaining the same line of direction (direction taking). The first is *squaring off*, so that one is perpendicular to an object or a wall surface.

SQUARING OFF AND DIRECTION TAKING
• When the student comes to the opening and realizes it is not a doorway, she then goes around the corner and places her back to the new wall without changing her initial line of direction. The instructor monitors to ensure that the backs of the student's head, shoulders, hips, and feet are square to and up against the surface and that she is facing directly forward (is perpendicular to that surface).
• The student uses the upper hand and forearm and/or the lower hand and alternate arm techniques and projects herself forward and away from the wall surface to the opposite side of the corridor. Meanwhile, the instructor ensures a straight and safe crossing by standing directly opposite the student and up against the opposite wall and asks her to come to his voice; he moves out of the student's way at the last moment and places his hand on the palm of the student's upper hand as it is about to make contact with the wall. By doing so, he allows the student to make contact with the wall gently, rather than to run into it abruptly.

ALIGNING AND DIRECTION TAKING
• As an alternative to squaring off, the student determines if she is parallel to the initial wall line that she has been trailing by fanning her trailing hand along the surface from waist height in front of her to waist height in back of her. She is determining that the wall does not feel as though it is crossing her midline either in front of her (indicating that she is facing the wall) or behind her (indicating that she is facing away from the wall). The instructor helps the student feel these relationships by purposely placing her so she slightly faces toward or away from the wall.
• The student repositions herself so she is parallel to the wall line and grasps the corner of the intersecting walls with the trailing hand, places her other arm in the

upper hand and arm position, and propels herself forward and away from the wall intersection to the intersection or wall on the opposite side.

When the student uses the aligning-to-a-wall procedure, the instructor ensures a safe and straight crossing in the same way he did for the squaring-off procedure. After practicing this procedure back and forth, the student uses the technique, when necessary, to negotiate routes. As she practices the crossings, the instructor need not stand directly in front of her. If she drifts away from the intended wall during the crossing, the instructor provides verbal feedback accordingly. The student learns to estimate the distance across the opening and makes adjustments by turning 90 degrees toward the proper direction, if she does not encounter the opposite side when she expects to. (This readjustment from a veer is critical to learn now because it will also be used later when crossing streets.)

SEARCHING PATTERNS
FOR LOCATING DROPPED OBJECTS

Like everyone else, when people with visual impairments drop objects, they may need to retrieve them. However, they need to find them without the benefit of sight. This searching process can be done in a systematic fashion, and the student now has the necessary skills to accomplish it. However, the instructor must first determine if the student has the necessary capability to localize the source of a sound and carry out the task.

Assessing the Student's Ability to Localize
the Source of a Sound

The student's ability to localize the sources of sounds can be assessed by using the following procedure:
- The student sits in a chair in an echo-free room with a hardwood or tile floor.
- The instructor silently places keys directly in front of the student's face, in front of each ear, over her head, behind and above her head, and to the right or left side and below the seat (in front of and behind her).
- The instructor jingles the keys briefly at each location, and the student points to them. (The student may need to have the instructor grasp her hand and have it touch the jingling keys to understand what she should be doing.) He stops jingling the keys when placing them in a different position and plane to avoid alerting the student where the keys are to be jingled next.

When assessing the student's ability to locate the source of a sound, the instructor looks for any indication of a hearing loss, especially if the student does not accurately point to the keys in any or all the positions. If a hearing loss is suspected, he refers the student for an audiological examination. However, first, he should make sure that the student is not simply suffering from a head cold or sinus problem that is temporarily impeding her hearing or that she does not have accurate pointing skills. In such a case, the instructor should postpone the assessment until the student is recovered or has learned to point. If an audiological examination determines that the student does, indeed, have a hearing loss, the instructor looks for consistencies in localizing the sound and helps the student make adjustments to determine more accurately where its source is located.

Locating Dropped Objects

Once it has been determined that the student can accurately localize the direction of a sound source, then the student can learn the skill necessary to recover objects that she may drop. The procedure is as follows:

- The student stands in an open area, and the instructor jingles some keys and drops them directly in front of the student and near her feet. The student squats, bending at the knees but not at the waist, while protecting her face using the upper hand and forearm technique. She then places both hands palm down and flat on the floor between her feet. She begins a fanning motion with her hands flat on the floor, searching the floor directly around and between her feet. She continues to scan the floor farther and farther away from her feet without losing her balance until she finds the keys.

- The student stands, and the instructor repeats the process by dropping the keys on each side of the student, behind her, and out away from the her. If the keys are not directly in front of the student, she turns to place the source of the sound directly in front of her and then begins to search. If the sound seems to be several feet away, the student turns to the sound and steps forward, underestimating the distance from the source before beginning the search. In this way, she does not risk stepping over the object and inadvertently placing it behind her. If she still does not find the object, she scoots forward a few steps while protecting herself before beginning the search pattern anew.

- The instructor incorporates a variety of objects for the student to find and chooses objects that make a sound when dropped and are large enough to be easily located. The student progresses to locating smaller and smaller objects and, finally, objects that roll. Easy objects to begin with are a set of keys, a notepad, a pen or pencil, and a comb or brush. More difficult objects to locate are coins, a ball, and a spool of thread.

- If a long cane is available, it can be used in the search process as follows: The student localizes the source of the sound and faces it. She stoops and places the cane on the ground directly in front of her with the tip pointing away from her. She gently grasps the cane grip with her thumb and first two fingers without lifting it off the ground and pivots the cane flat along the floor from right to left like a pendulum until she feels the cane come into contact with the object. She then traces along the cane shaft until she finds the object. This procedure works only with large objects that cannot slip into the space between the cane shaft and the grip as the cane is pivoted.

- If the student cannot stoop to search for objects that have fallen, she can use her feet, a broom, or some other object to sweep and fan to locate them.

CONSIDERATIONS FOR EFFECTIVE TEACHING

Using Exercises to Reinforce the Techniques

The instructor can reinforce the correct arm and hand positions for the upper hand and forearm technique by using the following isometric exercise: Standing in front of and facing the student, he asks the student to assume the correct position and then places his hand against the student's upper hand, palm to palm. The student then pushes her upper hand against the instructor's hand several times. This exercise can also be done to reinforce the lower hand and alternate arm technique by the instructor's pressing against the student's alternate arm when it is in the correct position, to integrate the feeling of the correct positions into the respective shoulder joints. The student practices placing her arm and hand in the correct positions, using either hand and arm, until she does so to the instructor's satisfaction. The student walks along the corridors and, at the instructor's request, varies which hand and arm are in the upper hand and forearm (or lower hand and alternate arm) position.

Learning Indoor Numbering Systems

The student learns that, as is the case with outdoor address systems, there is an order and logic to indoor numbering systems within a building even though indoor numbering systems vary from building to building. For instance, in some buildings odd numbers are on one side of a hall and even numbers are on the other side. Or, the numbers may run consecutively up one side of a hall and down the other side. Numbers from 1 to 99 may indicate the first floor of a building; 100 to 199, the second floor; and so on.

Although it is important to be able to discern a building's numbering system, it may not be practical to learn the number of every room on every floor. In an office building, for instance, the student may need to know only a particular floor and a particular side of the floor to look for a specific office because she will use a landmark on that side to locate the office. For example, she may know in advance that her dentist's office is located in room 201 and is one door away from a drinking fountain as she exits from the elevator. In this example, if she knows that the odd numbers are located on the east side of the hallways, then when she arrives on that floor she trails along the east side until she locates the water fountain and then trails to the next door, which should be her destination. In any event, if she is unsure, she can simply walk into an office and ask for assistance.

Working with Students with Low Vision

Although low vision students on occasion may make effective use of self-protection techniques, especially in dimly lighted or high-glare situations, these techniques may be more casually exhibited in the curriculum than they are for students without usable vision and may be implemented only occasionally or with modifications. For instance, the upper forearm may be held at waist height and still afford adequate protection. In general, instructors working with students with remaining vision need to ensure that the upper forearm position does not cover their students' eyes and hence does not block their vision. A student's needs and degree of vision loss help determine how that student will use a given technique. For example, a student with low vision may not need to hand trail a wall to locate a door, but may use the upper forearm procedure when approaching and walking through the doorway to ensure that she is protected from swinging doors. Another student may be able to see a table from a distance, but lose sight of it as she approaches it; therefore, she might use the alternate hand and arm procedure as she walks toward it.

Modifying the Sequence of Instruction

Depending on where the student is being taught the skills and her immediate needs, the sequence of instruction may have to be modified. If the student is taught at home, she may first need to learn to hand trail a wall to locate objects in the living room, since there may not be enough room to walk out into open spaces. In fact, it may be necessary to teach the student how to trail along the walls of her home before teaching most of the sighted guide procedures outlined in Chapter 3.

Knowing When to Move on

As the student learns a particular skill, the instructor notes how easily and naturally the student demonstrates the technique: Are the arms rigid? Is the free arm tense? Do the shoulders rise as the upper forearm position is demonstrated? Affirmative answers to these and other questions may indicate that the student is not yet ready to move on. However, over time the student will relax, and the procedures will become ingrained if the instructor allows her ample time to practice the techniques in a variety of situations. A student can move on to hand trailing even if she does not demonstrate smooth and coordinated upper forearm and hand positions in open spaces; since she will use this position when trailing, she will be practicing it as she learns to hand trail. Once again, it is preferable to overlearn a motor skill to ensure that it can be used in conjunction with other skills.

5

Basic Long Cane and Self-Familiarization Skills

The long cane is the most frequently used mode of travel for persons with visual impairments who travel by themselves and without the assistance of someone else. After learning to use the long cane and to familiarize themselves with various environments, students will be able to travel in a wide variety of situations independently and will in all likelihood use the cane in most travel situations in the future. This chapter explains how the student begins this process by learning the diagonal cane technique and how to become familiar with an unfamiliar room.

RIGID LONG CANES

It is important for the student to become familiar with the parts of a cane, the types of canes that are available, and the care and maintenance of the long cane. It is the instructor's responsibility to inform the student of the various options in choosing a long cane, the strengths and weaknesses of the various canes on the market, and how to take care of and maintain the cane.

As the student learns the cane skills, he will be responsible for handling the cane properly in various situations to ensure his safety and the safety of others. Therefore, the student is responsible for bringing the cane to each lesson, properly caring for it, and replacing parts as they wear out or break. He learns to respect what the cane can and cannot detect and that it signifies that one who uses it has some degree of visual impairment.

There are two basic types of long canes: rigid canes and folding canes. Rigid canes are generally used during lessons because they are more durable and provide greater sensory information than folding canes. Folding canes are often preferred by seasoned travelers because they are more portable and more easily disposed of when not needed than are rigid canes. The student learns to carry a spare folding cane with him when he is using a rigid cane for extended periods in case the latter bends or breaks during travel. (Folding canes will be described further in Chapter 10.)

The standard rigid long cane is made of aluminum; is hollow inside; and has a white nylon tip at one end. This cane has changed little since its development by Richard Hoover and his colleagues during World War II. Various adaptations of the standard rigid cane include canes made out of fiberglass with a metal glide tip, as the National Federation of the Blind (NFB)-made cane; canes without a crook; canes with an elastic cord on the grip end instead of the crook; canes without a crook or an elastic cord on the ends; and canes with a larger marshmallow or mushroom nylon tip. One recent development includes a cane with a long, U-shaped tip, the Bundu Basher cane, which is used in rural South Africa to travel along rugged terrain. Canes can be used with or without a coating of white-and-red reflective tape. For more information on suppliers and manufacturers of canes, see Gill (in press) and Sources of Long Canes in the Resources section.

Parts of the Long Cane

The long cane has four basic parts: the crook, with a plastic cap on the end to keep debris from entering the hollow shaft and to protect the user from getting cut on the crook edge; the rubber grip, which is made out of a golf putter grip that has a flat edge along one side on which the user places the index finger; the long aluminum shaft; and the cane tip, which is made out of hard nylon and slips either over or into the end of the shaft.

The crook. The crook is useful for hanging up the cane when it is not in use. It helps the user determine tactilely where to grasp the cane in that it points down to the ground when the cane is allowed to rest naturally in the hand. The crook is helpful when the cane does not have a grip with a flat side to position the index finger easily and protects the knuckles when the diagonal cane technique, described later in this chapter, is used. If the cane is accidentally dropped on a slope, moreover, the crook will ensure that it will not roll far away from the user.

The rubber grip. The rubber grip enables the user to grasp the cane in various temperatures and situations without losing control of it. The grip is unaffected by wide swings in temperature and protects the user's hand from perspiration in the heat and the shaft's coldness in low temperatures. The grip is glued or cemented onto the shaft, one end even with the crook edge, with the flat side either to the right or left side of the cane when the crook is pointing down to the ground. (The cane is considered a right-handed cane if the flat side is on the right and a left-handed cane if it is on the left side.) If there is no crook, the same cane can be prescribed equally for right- handed or left-handed users.

The long shaft. The aluminum shaft is covered by red and/or white strips of reflective tape. The strips have heat-sensitive backings that, when heat friction is induced, will bond the tape with the aluminum and provide a protective coating for the shaft. The colors identify a traveler with a visual impairment to the seeing public, which is especially helpful when the person is entering potentially dangerous situations or asking for assistance. The red strip is five inches long and is positioned along the shaft just above the edge of the cane tip. The white strip extends along the shaft from the edge of the red strip to the grip; its length depends on the remaining length of the shaft after the red strip is applied. If the cane is manufactured without the strips, the instructor usually applies the strips after the student has learned to handle and care for the cane for some time during the O&M program and just before he needs to ask for assistance from the public.

The tip. The hard nylon tip is long and narrow and conducts sensory information about the terrain on which the user is walking. It wears down over time and is replaced before it reaches the shaft. If the cane is held consistently and properly, the tip should wear down along the under edge when the two-point-touch technique is used. As it wears, the tip should glide more easily along the ground.

Marshmallow, mushroom, and teardrop-shaped tips are round (or more oval) and smaller in length than is the standard nylon tip and fit just over the end of the shaft. These tips add weight to the end of the cane, which can aid people who have difficulty feeling the cane tip on the ground (such as elderly students or those with diabetes who lack feeling in their hands because of poor blood circulation). These tips also glide more easily on various surfaces and thus are the tips preferred by many instructors and cane users, especially those who have multiple impairments.

Measuring, Assembling, and Storing the Long Cane

It is the responsibility of the O&M instructor to prescribe the type of cane to be used in lessons and to measure the student for a cane of the proper length, taking into consideration a number of variables. When she issues the cane, the instructor may have to assemble the various parts on the aluminum shaft. Normally, canes can be purchased completely assembled; however, some agencies and schools still maintain a number of unassembled cane shafts. It is important, therefore, for the instructor to be familiar with the procedures for assembling a long rigid cane if she needs to do so.

MEASURING THE CANE

The determination of the initial length of the cane is somewhat arbitrary at this point in the student's program, but the length will be close to the eventual prescribed length. Other factors will eventually determine the exact length. For example, later the instructor will note the length of the student's stride, the student's reaction time to locating obstacles in his path, and the student's ability to detect drop-offs. As the student relaxes as he uses the cane during the next focus of instruction, outdoor residential travel, the instructor observes the student's foot and cane placements while he walks along a sidewalk. She notes whether the student's cane tip touches down where his foot will be placed next. If the student over- or understeps the cane, the cane will have to be cut down or a new, longer cane prescribed, accordingly. Therefore, it is recommended that the instructor measure the cane slightly longer than is described next because it is easier to cut more off the cane than to add more onto it. The initial length is measured as follows:

- With the student standing erect, the instructor places a cane on its crook or grip end, vertically to the ground, up against the student's midline and with the tip end resting on the student's chest.
- The cane is marked where it touches the base of the student's sternum; two inches are added to this mark; and a new line is marked, which is where the cane will be cut. As an alternative, the instructor marks the cane where it touches the base of the student's armpit, which usually is two inches higher from the ground than is the measurement from the base of the sternum.
- Using a tube cutter, the instructor cuts off the excess shaft along the marked line and sands down the sharp edge.

ASSEMBLING THE CANE

After the desired length has been measured and cut, the cane can be assembled. The grip is assembled first. It can be purchased at most golf-pro shops and is hollow inside and open at its bottom end.

- A hole, corresponding in diameter to the open end, is cut out of its closed top end with a knife.
- A small, quarter-inch-thick block of plywood is used to push the grip onto the shaft. To do so, a hole is drilled into the center of the block slightly larger than the diameter of the cane shaft but smaller than the diameter of the grip.
- The cane is placed into a vise at the crook end with the crook facing down. Care should be taken to wrap the crook with a towel or other cloth to avoid damaging it with the vise.
- A lubricant, like liquid dishwashing detergent, is applied to the shaft to make it easier to slide the grip along the shaft.
- Glue is poured into the grip, and the grip is slid onto the tip end of the shaft with the top of the grip closest to the crook. The shaft sticks out somewhat beyond the bottom of the grip, so the block of wood can be inserted onto the shaft.
- The block of wood is then used to push the grip up the shaft into position. The grip is positioned so that its top is just below the end of the crook and the flat side is along the desired side of the shaft.
- The excess lubricant and glue are wiped off the shaft, the shaft is cleaned with rubbing alcohol, and the glue in the grip is allowed to dry overnight.
- After the glue has dried, the plastic cap is inserted on the end of the crook. Grips can be inserted directly on the grip end of canes that have no crooks.

To install the tip, the instructor first determines if the tip is to be placed over the shaft or into the shaft. (Tips that mount over the shaft may have to be boiled and then frozen and thawed to make them pliable enough to get on over the shaft.)

- Once the tip can be eased onto the shaft by hand, the instructor gently taps it down further by tapping it on the ground until it sits firmly, is straight, and is as far as it can go on the end of the shaft.

Tips that are inserted into the shaft have a piece of rubber slipped between a slit into the thin end that is inserted into the shaft. It is important to leave this rubber in the slit because it allows for the expansion and contraction of the tip in various temperatures and thus helps to keep the tip securely in place. This type of tip is installed as follows:

- The instructor inserts the tip into the shaft as much as possible, and then turns the cane over and lightly taps the tip on the ground and into the cane, until it is seated firmly in place.

The reflective strips are applied in the following manner:

- The red strip is applied first. The instructor cuts a five-inch strip of red tape from a roll of Scotchlite reflective tape.
- With the cane held in one hand by the grip and the tip facing up and away from her, the instructor rubs the shaft with a cloth or paper towel on the spot to which the strip will be applied to create heat friction.
- After the instructor feels a buildup of heat, she places the cane flat on a table with the flat side of the grip facing up and the tip to her right. She then removes the backing of the strip and carefully places the strip lengthwise along the shaft with one edge centered lengthwise on the center of the shaft and one edge almost touching the end of the cane tip. (If the grip has been placed properly, there is a thin white line that runs down the middle of the flat edge of the grip that can be used to determine the center of the shaft when applying the strip of reflective tape.)
- The instructor then picks up the cane by the grip with one hand and uses the other hand to press the strip onto the shaft. She uses the towel to press against the strip that is attached to the shaft and rubs up and down the strip on the shaft while slowly rotating the cane. She is careful not to let the strip fold or bubble because it is not possible to pull the strip off once it adheres to the cane. Once the strip has been rubbed in place, the seam is on the bottom side of the cane when the crook is facing down.
- The white strip is then applied in a similar manner: It is cut to extend along the shaft from the edge of the red strip to just before the end of the grip. Because of its length, the white strip is more difficult to apply. Care must be taken to align its edge properly and evenly lengthwise and to rub it on evenly with the towel. If the white strip is applied correctly, its seam will be aligned with the red strip's seam so that one long seam will be apparent from the underside of the cane and will not be seen when viewed from any of the sides when the cane is in use.

After both strips are applied properly, the cane appears to be coated with the red and white colors and none of the aluminum is visible, except on the crook. The cane is now fully assembled.

STORING THE CANE

The cane can be propped up against a wall or laid on the floor, flat up against and parallel to a wall. If the cane has a crook or elastic loop, it can be hooked on to the top edge of an open door or on to a coat hook, hat rack, or hanger rod. In all cases, the student must find locations that do not interfere with traffic, are safe to traverse without the cane, and can be easily found when the cane is desired.

THE SIGHTED GUIDE TECHNIQUE WITH A LONG CANE

Once the cane is initially fitted and assembled for the student, the instructor shows the student how to use it while walking with a sighted guide. The student uses the cane with a guide in one of three ways: (1) he learns to keep it out of the way during the procedures; (2) he learns to use it in a diagonal fashion after he learns the diagonal cane skills, as described later in this chapter; or (3) he learns to use it while using the two-point-touch technique, described in Chapter 6. The latter two ways are learned after the respective cane skills are thoroughly understood. The initial lessons using the cane with sighted guide skills are accomplished with the cane held out of the way, or in the "not-in-use" position, as follows:

Basic sighted guide position. In the basic sighted guide position, the student holds the cane in his free hand with the fingers and thumb wrapped around the grip (or just below the grip on the shaft), slightly in front of him and off to the side. The arm holding the cane is bent at the elbow, and the cane is held vertically to the ground.

Turns and reversing directions. When the instructor and student pivot around each other in turning and reversing directions, the cane is held in the not-in-use manner. To reverse directions using the about-face procedure, the two turn to face each other. The student places the cane in the hand that is holding on to the instructor. He places the cane vertically to the ground and flat against the instructor's arm, with the cane between the palm (or thumb) and the guiding arm. The student finds the instructor's free arm with the freed hand of the "cane" arm. He lets go of the original arm and grasps the cane in the not-in-use position. As he grasps the instructor's new guiding arm in the basic sighted guide position, they turn to face in the opposite direction (see Figures 5.1-5.3).

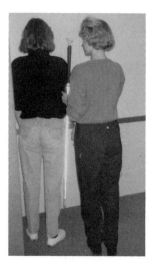
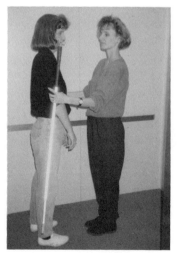
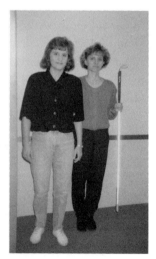

Figures 5.1-5.3 Executing the about-face procedure while holding a cane and entering an elevator.

Narrow spaces. The cane is held as described in the basic sighted guide position.

Transferring sides. While the instructor and student are transferring sides, the cane is switched to the instructor's guiding arm and the student's hand is run across the instructor's back until it finds the instructor's other guiding arm; the newly freed hand locates the instructor's new guiding arm and grasps it while the cane hand lets go of the arm.

Walking through doors that are initially closed. As the instructor and student walk through doors together, the student transfers the cane into the hand of the instructor's guiding arm before grasping the door edge, closes the door behind them, and then transfers the cane back into the original cane hand.

On stairs. When using a handrail on the side of the cane hand, the student places the cane against the instructor's guiding arm while grasping the arm; if the handrail is on the instructor's side or if there is no handrail, the student maintains the not-in-use position (or one of the diagonal cane positions, described later).

Seating. When the student takes a seat, the cane is placed underneath a couch or chair, so it is out of the way of other persons who may be seated or walking nearby. The student places one or both feet on the cane to ensure that it is not inadvertently kicked away from him. As an alternative, the student places the cane diagonally to the ground with the shaft in between his legs and the tip between his feet and rests the grip up against one shoulder (or vertically to the ground). He holds on to the shaft with one or both hands. When seating himself at a table, the student places the cane in the hand holding on to the table, so when he pulls out the chair, he is free to clear the chair of objects before sitting on it.

Hines break. If someone attempts to grab the student by the arm of the cane hand, the student quickly transfers the cane into the other hand and slips the crook or elastic cord between the thumb and the index finger. He lets the cane hang while he initiates the procedure and grasps the person's wrist with the new cane hand to break the individual's grasp. At the same time, he either politely rejects the offer for assistance and disengages himself from the person or accepts the assistance and grasps the individual's arm in the basic sighted guide position with his newly freed hand. If someone grasps the student's free arm (the one not holding the cane), the student initiates the procedure just described, but without transferring the cane into the other hand.

Auditoriums. When entering an auditorium, the student keeps the cane in the not-in-use position and ensures that it does not come into contact with other persons as he and the guide walk together down the aisle and into the rows.

Cafeterias. When the student is obtaining food in a cafeteria, the cane is held as described in Chapter 3. As an alternative to holding the cane under the armpit when carrying a tray, the student can hook the crook of the cane on the back of his collar or on his shirt, just above the top button. In these ways the cane is kept out of the way and he is free to carry his tray with both hands.

THE DIAGONAL CANE TECHNIQUE

The diagonal cane technique is the first of two basic cane techniques used for independent travel. It enhances the student's ability to travel independently through a familiar indoor environment. The second cane technique, the two-point-touch technique (described in detail in Chapter 6), enables the student to travel in all types of situations, both familiar and unfamiliar. Each technique can be performed with various modifications that are appropriate in different travel situations and conditions. In the case of the diagonal cane technique, the student learns when to implement all the diagonal cane procedures and is given enough time to practice each one sufficiently. The diagonal cane technique is useful in familiar indoor areas because with it, the student detects many known objects or obstacles but does not adequately detect objects encountered outside the areas of cane protection or areas with drop-offs (in which the level of the walking surface drops off to a lower level, such as on a descending stairway or from a curb into a street). Therefore, the student must learn these limitations and exercise caution when traveling even in familiar indoor areas. Even familiar areas can change from moment to moment and day to day: Buckets and ladders can be placed along well-known hallways temporarily when construction work, painting, or even cleaning is being done. Using the diagonal cane technique, the student could easily have his cane go under the ladder without contacting it and could cause himself serious injury.

Although the cane technique has its limitations, it still offers more protection than do self-protection techniques. The cane acts as a bumper for the body and a buffer between the body and obstacles in the environment. Because the cane also identifies its user as having a visual impairment, people who are traveling in hallways while lessons are being conducted may have a tendency to move out of the student's way, which can be helpful or detrimental, depending on the goals of the lessons.

The student first learns to hold the cane while in the various sighted guide positions, as described earlier. The instructor determines whether the student will then be introduced to all the diagonal cane grasps or to just one or two of them. Her decision will be determined, in part, by her knowledge of the student's ability to grasp with his fingers; any physical impairments in the hands, arms, and shoulders; and the student's ability to use previously learned motor skills. Thus, if the student had difficulty rotating his wrist and shoulder as he learned to trail with his arm, the instructor may decide not to teach him to use the index finger grasp, which places a good deal of stress on the wrist, elbow, and shoulder. If it is necessary for the student to use the index finger grasp, the instructor can modify the technique to meet the physical requirements of her student.

The same indoor environment selected for the lesson on self-protection techniques should suffice for lessons on the diagonal cane technique. Hallways that are uncluttered are excellent areas to introduce walking with a sighted guide while holding a cane and the initial diagonal cane lessons. As the student learns the skills, he travels through areas with more hallway furniture and through congested rooms to practice the skills while manipulating the cane in and around the obstacles.

Types of Grasps

THE INDEX FINGER GRASP

The basic grasp for implementing the diagonal cane technique, the index finger grasp, is positioned as follows:

- The instructor faces the student, whose back is against a wall, and places the cane into the student's dominant hand as if the student were shaking hands with the cane and with the midpoint of the grip flat against the center of the palm. The student places the index finger along the flat side with the other fingers and thumb wrapped around the grip.
- The student then rotates the wrist of his cane hand inward or toward him, so his palm is facing somewhat away from him and the cane is placed diagonally across his body.
- The cane arm is extended directly forward and away from the body to arm's length. If there is a crook, it is wrapped around the knuckles and projects away from the student.
- The cane tip touches the floor approximately two inches beyond the widest portion of the body (see Figure 5.4).

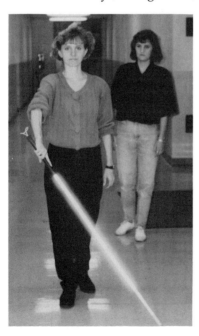

Figure 5.4 The index finger grasp of the diagonal cane technique.

When viewed from the front, the cane appears to be diagonally across the student's body, extending two inches beyond the shoulder of the dominant side to two inches beyond the opposite shoulder. In this position, the cane will act as a bumper for objects below the waist and in the student's way as he moves through the environment. Many students have difficulty feeling that the cane is diagonally across the body and often think that the cane arm is not positioned forward but off to the dominant side. The instructor helps the student understand this relationship to his body by grasping the cane as it is held properly in position and by allowing the student to let go of it entirely to run both hands along the cane shaft. The student then "feels" the diagonal nature of the technique as he glides his hands along the shaft from the grip on the dominant side to the tip on the nondominant side. In addition, the instructor performs an isometric exercise in which the student, while the cane is in position, presses his cane hand toward his midline and against the instructor's hand, so he feels the correct positioning in the shoulder of his dominant side. The student practices grasping the cane and extending it properly in a stationary posture before moving into an open space.

THE THUMB GRASP

The second diagonal cane grasp is called the thumb grasp. It is positioned as follows:

- All the fingers are wrapped around the grip with the thumb pointing down toward the tip and against the flat side of the grip.
- The hand and arm positions are the same as for the index finger grasp.
- The same exercises and procedures are used for both grasps.

THE PENCIL GRASP

The third diagonal cane grasp is called the pencil grasp and is positioned as follows:

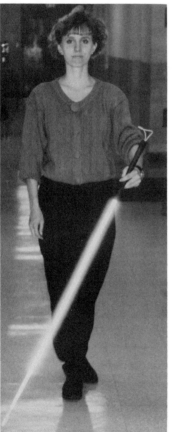

Figure 5.5 The pencil grasp of the diagonal cane technique.

- The student grasps the cane with the grip placed between the thumb and the index finger. The thumb and index finger are wrapped around the grip, and the remaining fingers are cupped together and used to counterbalance the cane from underneath.
- The cane is pointed diagonally across the body with the tip touching the floor approximately two inches beyond the opposite shoulder. The cane hand is held either forward with the arm at arm's length from the student or forward with the arm bent at the elbow and with the elbow braced against the student's rib cage (see Figure 5.5). The student learns to feel the correct position in the elbow and shoulder of the dominant side by performing the following isometric exercise with the instructor: While in position, the student presses his cane hand toward his midline and against the instructor's hand, relaxes it, and repeats the procedure several times.

The sequence of the lesson should move from simple motor skills to more complex skills. One skill should be learned well before another is added. Therefore, the instructor does not introduce all the grasps in the same lesson, but gives the student time to practice each sufficiently in either hand and with the tip of the cane on or off the floor. While using any of the three grasps, the student keeps his free arm relaxed at his side or in the upper hand and forearm technique. The instructor observes the free arm to ensure that it is relaxed while the student moves into open spaces. At first, the student will probably hold the free arm stiffly as he concentrates on positioning the cane hand and arm. As he learns the skills, his free arm should relax and swing normally at his side.

Walking into Open Spaces

Lessons progress from travel in open spaces to trailing and then to a mix of each—similar to the sequence described for self-protection techniques in Chapter 4. The student learns to walk forward into open spaces maintaining the proper positioning of each grasp while following the instructor's voice. Before he learns another grasp, he learns one grasp well with one hand and then learns to use it with the other hand. Finally, he learns to switch grasps in either hand while in motion. When the cane grasps are switched within each hand and between hands, the cane is not lifted off the ground more than one or two inches. The cane is allowed to glide along the ground and later to remain lifted off the ground one or two inches while in motion.

By the end of this mini-unit of instruction, the student should be able to walk down a hallway and change grasps at will. He should know when to use each grasp and how to manipulate the cane to assume any of the grasps in either hand. For example, he learns that the index finger grasp affords the best control when trailing a wall and that the thumb grasp is especially useful when walking into open spaces where there is little pedestrian traffic because the cane position is easily maintained and maneuvered. However, when many people are present, the pencil grasp may allow him to manipulate the cane in and around their feet gently as they stand or walk by. Ultimately, the student decides which cane grasp to use and when, since all students have their own preferences for certain grasps.

Contacting and Examining Objects

As the student makes contact with the wall at the end of the hallway with his cane at the end of a route, he positions the cane tip up against the wall while rotating his cane hand inward. He approaches the wall so the cane shaft becomes vertical to the ground and is at his midline. He then turns around and places his back to the wall to indicate he has completed the route. When he contacts an object that is below the cane grip, he follows the same procedure but takes his free hand and runs it down the shaft to contact and then explore the object. To avoid losing his balance while exploring, he squats without leaning forward as he runs his hand down along the shaft to find the object. After he learns to find and explore objects to identify them, the student is encouraged to explore and identify objects only when necessary, because this practice slows down his travel and diverts his attention from other more important environmental cues in more advanced travel situations later in the program.

Trailing a Wall while Using the Diagonal Technique

After the student learns to use diagonal cane skills while walking into open spaces, he learns to use each grasp while trailing a wall line. Each grasp is practiced first while the cane is in the student's dominant hand and then in the nondominant hand. Therefore, the student walks along a wall with the cane in the dominant hand, and then the instructor walks back along the wall with the student in the sighted guide position to repractice the procedure with the cane in the dominant hand. After many trips along the wall in this manner, the instructor introduces the skill in the nondominant hand. The student is brought back to the starting point using the sighted guide technique after each trip. Once he practices the skill numerous times in both hands, the student then practices walking along the wall back and forth with the cane in the appropriate hand each time (see Figure 5.6).

Trailing a wall with no objects or openings. To trail a wall in which there are no openings or protruding objects, the student stands parallel to the wall with the nondominant shoulder nearly touching the wall. He holds the cane in the index finger grasp with the tip touching the wall and slightly off the floor. The student maintains the proper position while trailing along the wall with the cane tip, preferably using a light touch. He may choose to keep his free arm at his side or in his pocket, bent at the elbow and across the small of his back, or in the upper hand and forearm position.

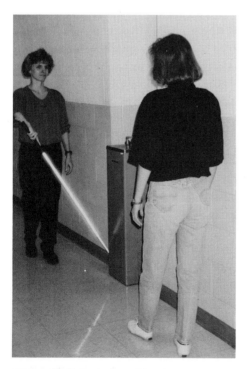

Figure 5.6 The index finger grasp of the diagonal cane technique, used in conjunction with trailing a wall.

Trailing across doorways or corridors. In trailing across openings in a wall, such as doorways or corridors, when the student's cane tip contacts a door jamb or end of a wall line, it is projected forward and parallel to the wall as the student moves forward across the opening. The tip will contact the opposite door jamb or wall after the student's cane has crossed the opening. Care is taken not to allow the tip to be pushed into the opening, so the cane does not bang into closed doors or trip anyone in the doorway or corridor or get hung up in the opening. The student learns to avoid these problems by performing a slight arching motion away from and back toward the wall as the tip crosses the opening. Finally, the student learns to distinguish doorways from corridors by the length and time it takes to make the crossing: doorway crossings are generally shorter than are corridor crossings.

SELF-FAMILIARIZATION SKILLS: THE ROOM-FAMILIARIZATION PROCEDURE

The lessons on the room-familiarization procedure are the first to put the onus of learning the environment directly on the student. As the student gains sighted guide, self-protection, and some basic cane skills, he is concurrently developing rudimentary orientation skills. Until this point, however, he has moved through the environment with his instructor's guidance and tutelage and hence has not had to understand fully all the intricacies of the building in which he has received instruction. As he learns the room-familiarization procedure, he will discover the basics of acquainting himself with any room or floor of a building, an entire building, or any outdoor travel area. Therefore, the instructor should help the student to learn this procedure thoroughly and to transfer the skill to numerous other environments.

To teach the self-familiarization process, the instructor first uses a small room containing only a few pieces of furniture. After the student has used the procedure, he explores rooms containing a variety of types of furniture, shapes, and configurations to determine if the skill can be transferred to other unfamiliar environments. The instructor observes the student during these later lessons and provides less and less verbal feedback while the student explores the areas.

The student's transfer of skills to other rooms can be documented in several ways. First, the student can be asked to walk through a room and to point out its various characteristics. Second, the student can make a tactile or low vision map of the room to demonstrate knowledge of its contents. Third, the student can make an auditory map of the room. Obviously, the student first has to learn how to make these maps. As a general rule, the instructor does not expect her students to be able to do what they have not yet been taught. This rule of thumb is applied to every situation in which the student interacts with the environment and guides the instructor's determination of when to intervene during a lesson. If the student has not yet experienced a situation that occurs in a lesson, the instructor should not expect him to use acceptable skills or procedures. The instructor judges whether to intercede or not, and if so, when and how. These decisions are the core to guiding the student toward independent travel skills.

The room-familiarization procedure is usually introduced after the instructor judges that the student has gained the necessary requisite skills. Because the room is "unfamiliar" to the student, technically the student should already have learned the two-point-touch cane technique, since this skill is the first in which the student will be adequately protected while moving through an unfamiliar environment. However, the instructor may wish to introduce the process before the student has learned any cane skills but has adequate self-protection skills if the instructor thinks the cane would only get in the way at first. The room-familiarization procedure applies to any room and is learned in the sequence of perimeter familiarization and the use of the grid pattern that follows.

Perimeter Familiarization

Room familiarization begins with exploration of a room's perimeter in the following way:

- The instructor guides the student into the room and closes the door behind them, and the student places his back to the closed door. The instructor explains the reasons for learning to become familiar with a room and the procedures that will be followed.

- The student uses the door through which he entered the room as his home base, or *reference point*, because it is the only known component of the room as yet. He then explores the door with his hands to find recognizable features, since there may be numerous other doors in the room and he must be able to discern his home base from the other doors. Therefore, he explores the door frame, jambs, and knobs or push bars; searches for windows or other identifiable markings; and identifies the material from which the door is made. He then explores right next to the door for light switches or any other identifying characteristics.

- With his back again to the door, the student determines the true compass directions. If they are unknown, it is possible for the sake of this procedure to use contrived compass directions until the true ones are known. That is, the student can arbitrarily decide that north will be in front of him with his back to the door and thus home base will be on the "south" wall. For the sake of the rest of the description of this procedure, it is assumed that the reference door is on the south wall. After the student has explored the walls, he can decide to name them after some distinguishing landmark; for instance, the south wall could be called the "door wall" if there are no other doors in the room or "wall 1" if the student has difficulty using cardinal directions.

- The student trails along the south wall from one end to the other, always returning to the reference door before exploring farther into the room. He begins to catalog in his mind or on audiotape the location of furniture, bulletin boards, blackboards, windows, and whatever else he finds along the wall and the order in which he finds them.

- The student begins exploring other walls, one at a time, always retracing his steps back to the reference-point door. For example, he travels from the door to the east wall (in the southeastern corner of the room), and trails the east wall north until he finds the north wall (in the northeastern corner of the room). He then retraces his route back along the east wall south to the southeastern corner and along the south wall to the door.

- He then trails back along the east wall to the north wall, turns west, and trails to the west wall (in the northwestern corner of the room). He reverses the route back along the north and east walls to the door.

- He follows this process until he has thoroughly explored all the walls in the room (see Figure 5.7). He then points to various objects along the walls from his reference point to show that he understands the relationships of the objects to each other and to the reference point.

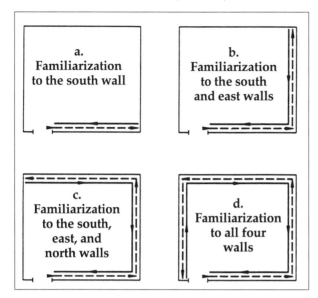

Figure 5.7 Perimeter room-familiarization procedure.

• He walks routes to and from various objects along the walls and occasionally points to objects in the room from different reference points. His ability to do so shows the instructor (and the student) that he has begun to develop a mental or cognitive map of the room.

Having the student always retrace his steps back to the reference door accomplishes several things simultaneously. First, it gives the student the opportunity to come in contact with the numerous objects along the wall many times, so their locations will less likely have to be memorized. Second, objects missed for whatever reasons will probably be contacted after several trips along the wall. Third, the trailing skills are reinforced in practical situations, and motor skills are paired with cognitive skills. And fourth, the student learns that he is never in jeopardy of losing his orientation if he always returns to his familiar home base after branching out into unfamiliar territory.

After thoroughly learning about the walls of the room, the student is now ready to explore the room's interior. As he does so, he learns three things about the room. First, he learns about the objects in the room's center. Second, he reaffirms the relationship of objects along the walls; that is, he learns which objects are, indeed, opposite each other on opposite walls. And third, he reaffirms the shape of the room by walking in the open space to opposite walls by using the following procedure.

The Grid Pattern

After the perimeter of a room is explored, the grid pattern is used by the student to explore the center of the room. The grid pattern is used in the following way:

• With his back to the door, the student squares off, protects himself, and crosses from the south wall to the north wall. To facilitate a straight crossing, the instructor has the student come to her voice at first. If there are any objects in the student's path, he explores them, goes around them, and continues on his way across the room.

• Upon reaching the north wall, the student puts his back to and squares off with the wall and faces south. He then takes several steps either to his east or west, depending on the location of the reference door, and crosses back over to the south wall.

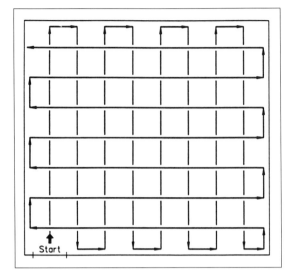

Figure 5.8 Grid pattern of the room-familiarization procedure.

• He continues this procedure either easterly or westerly until he has crossed over the entire width of the room. He may choose to follow the same procedure going north or south along the east and west walls until an imaginary grid pattern has been formed with the "lines" of his route, as illustrated in Figure 5.8.

On completing the grid pattern, the student should be completely familiar with the configuration of the room and all the objects in it. As he explores, he will occasionally locate numerous objects along the walls and at the center. When trailing the walls, if he encounters many objects along a wall, he may erroneously conclude that the wall is longer than its opposite counterpart in that it takes him longer to negotiate it than the other, which may have fewer objects. It is hoped that he can correctly judge the lengths of the walls when he implements the grid-pattern procedure and is able to walk an entire length of a wall unobstructed.

If the student encounters objects in the center of the room, he must negotiate them while maintaining the desired direction of travel. He can do so by pretending to "walk through" an object. For instance, if he encounters a rectangular table in front of him, he first explores it to determine where along that table he is and then trails to its opposite side, squares off to it, and continues crossing forward until he locates the opposite wall. The instructor teaches him how to do so and provides verbal feedback as he attempts to do it on his own thereafter. He may actually encounter the table during many trips across the room. In each instance, he trails around it in the same direction each time (from the familiar to the unfamiliar). Round tables, however, are more difficult to "walk through" than are rectangular tables. At first, the instructor can stand at the opposite side of a round (or rectangular) table and have the student come to her voice as he trails to develop a kinesthetic memory of the experience for later use.

CONSIDERATIONS FOR EFFECTIVE TEACHING

Readiness for Cane Skills

Out of necessity, some students (such as those who live in rural areas and need to travel a dirt path to get to their mailboxes) may have to be taught how to use a cane early in their O&M program. Not only will they need to learn the two-point-touch cane technique (see Chapter 6) before they learn the diagonal cane procedure, but they may need to learn it outdoors before they master it indoors, as suggested. If a student is learning the sequence as suggested in the subsequent chapters of this text, he should be ready for cane skills upon demonstrating smooth and efficient self-protection procedures as he trails along walls and walks into open spaces and as he becomes familiar with rooms in a building. Some instructors prefer to teach the room-familiarization procedure as a culminating experience before they teach the cane techniques because the cane often gets in the way of objects in the room and can become a burden.

PRECANE DEVICES

As children with visual impairments grow and move about their immediate environments, instructors must decide when to introduce the use of canes. Preschoolers can be introduced to the notion of using a cane as a bumper and protector by learning to use precane devices. In the past few years, these devices have been fashioned out of plastic conduits or pipes to form a T–shape, with the stem, or the shaft, placed on the ground or floor so the child pushes it in front of him. Other devices form a rectangle of plastic pipes with a roller placed over the base for ease of movement. After the children learn to use these devices, and as their developmental levels allow, they may be ready to maneuver and manipulate a long cane especially cut for their height. Some instructors have taught children as young as 5 years old to use a cane.

LOW VISION CANE USERS

Individuals with low vision may need to use canes for identification when they cross streets or use public transportation, or they may need to rely on them in dimly lighted areas or in glare. Some instructors prefer to blindfold these students to teach them how to rely on canes, while others believe that blindfolding does not simulate poor lighting conditions and that the only true way to simulate the lighting conditions is to teach their students at night. Low vision simulators, especially those that block out the inferior visual field, are excellent tools to use when teaching cane skills because the students cannot look down at their canes while walking, but they can look forward to use their vision. Although the prognosis for some students may be poor, that is, it is likely that they will lose more or all their remaining vision some day, one cannot prepare them for the eventual loss of vision by blindfolding them and teaching the skills as if they were totally blind. Once the blindfold is removed, they will use whatever remaining vision they may have. Therefore, instructors are encouraged to work with the usable vision and, if it fluctuates or decreases permanently, make any adaptations or modifications based on their students' current visual status.

RELUCTANT CANE USERS

Some students may be technically ready to learn to use a cane but may not be ready emotionally. They may believe that there is a stigma attached to using a cane, especially if they have not adequately dealt with the loss of their vision. Some believe they can travel without a cane because they are "doing just fine" around their homes or schools. As instructors work with these students and get to know them as individuals, the rapport they develop should lead to trust between them. In subsequent lessons, the instructors broach the subject of using a cane and what it can do for the students. Some students may relent and agree to learn to use the cane while not being committed psychologically to it. Instructors will note that these students do not use their canes between lessons, forget to bring their canes to lessons, or have many excuses for not using them during lessons. Instructors should be patient with these students and encourage them over time. Lots of praise, developing meaningful experiences, relating the use of the cane to future situations important to the students, and peer pressure are all ways to encourage reluctant students to use canes.

Cane Manipulations with the Diagonal Cane Technique

As the student travels using the diagonal cane technique, the cane tip and shaft will occasionally stick into hallway furniture and open doorways, and he must extract the cane from these obstacles without damaging it and while protecting himself. To extract the cane, the student gently removes the tip or shaft from the object, maintains his line of direction, and keeps the cane in front of him when he reassumes the correct positioning. For example, as the student trails in a hallway along a wall on his left side and makes cane contact with the side of a bench against the wall, he turns 90 degrees away from the wall and trails along the side of the bench until his cane locates one of the front legs. He extracts the cane tip from underneath the bench. He then turns back 90 degrees so the bench is still on his left side and trails its front until he locates the opposite side with the cane tip, extracts the tip, and turns 90 degrees toward the wall and trails the side until he locates the wall with the cane. He extracts the tip from the rear leg and then turns 90 degrees to the right and continues trailing the wall in the desired direction. In this example, the student keeps the diagonal cane position throughout the many turns and while he extracts the tip from underneath the bench before each turn. In this manner, he learns always to maintain the correct position and, hence, he always has adequate protection.

Cane Clues

As the student maneuvers the cane through the environment, he learns to identify objects by touching them with the cane. He begins to extend his finger tips out farther into the environment through the cane shaft to the cane tip itself. The shaft and tip become extensions of his hand and fingers. Later, he will learn to extend even farther out into the environment auditorily and will rely less upon objects he contacts with his cane. For the present, he learns to identify objects without touching them with his hands. At first, he stops to explore an object with the cane, but as he gains skill, he learns to do so while in motion by observing where the cane contacted the object, the sound the object made as it was contacted by the cane, and the approximate dimensions of the object by noting where along the shaft he felt the opposing force of the object as the cane maneuvered along its surfaces.

Correction of Veering

As the student walks out using the diagonal cane technique, he adjusts his line of direction as he contacts objects in his path. For example, if he veers into the wall while walking into open spaces, he learns to turn slightly away from the wall and to continue walking. After a few paces, he will be in the center of the hall, where he turns again slightly toward the wall he contacted, which should realign him to face directly down the corridor. The instructor shows the student how to do so by standing behind him and gently holding on to his shoulders as he contacts the wall. She then guides the student slightly away from the wall, and when they reach the middle of the hallway, she realigns him to face the proper direction. The instructor continues this procedure as she observes the student veering into the wall until the student executes it on his own. Instructors should forewarn students who do not wish to be touched or are tactilely defensive before they lightly touch the students' shoulders or should describe in detail what needs to be done. Instructors may have to develop activities to lessen the tactile defensiveness of these students and can work closely with other professionals involved in the educational or rehabilitation process to overcome these difficulties.

The student takes care not to sidestep away from the wall because doing so will not alter his direction. Rather, sidestepping causes the student to make contact with the same wall a few paces farther along the route.

If the student wishes to check his relative location in the hallway, he can do so by sweeping the cane along the floor in a 90-degree arc from his midline to the side of his cane hand and then placing the cane into his other hand and repeating the procedure. It is important for the student not to cross his midline when sweeping to explore the ground surface because he may inadvertently turn his body to do so, which could then change his direction and alignment—an especially critical problem when standing at the intersection of two hallways, two sidewalks, or even two streets.

Generally, students tend to turn too far from the wall after encountering it, which only causes them to contact the opposite wall after a few paces. This "pinballing" effect—that is, the experience of bouncing from wall to wall—can be disconcerting to the student and should be eliminated as quickly as possible.

When trailing the wall line using the diagonal cane technique, the student will encounter open doorways and intersecting halls. To cross these openings he uses the same squaring off or aligning procedures described in Chapter 4. The student is careful not to stick the cane into the open space unless he can determine that there are no pedestrians attempting to cross his path. Once he is certain that the path is clear, he assumes the cane position and crosses the opening accordingly. It is advisable for the student to use the upper hand and forearm technique while crossing to make contact with objects that the cane does not detect.

Route Patterns

As the student gains familiarity with the diagonal cane technique, he walks various routes in the hallways while maintaining his orientation and proper cane manipulations. The same route patterns and sequencing are used as were described in earlier chapters. The instructor stands or walks farther away from the student as he travels along the route and provides feedback only when the cane skill is done incorrectly. By the end of the mini-unit, feedback from the instructor should be at a minimum during the routes because too much feedback can lead to the student's dependence on the instructor. At this point, the student should begin to determine at the end of each route whether he used the skills properly.

Room Familiarization

The room-familiarization technique can be introduced at several points within the curriculum, depending on the instructor's desires and the student's needs and skill level. It can be learned, for instance, immediately after hand trailing has been introduced and learned, in order to avoid having the student manipulate the cane in and around objects in the room. As an alternative, it can be introduced after diagonal cane skills are learned as a way of reinforcing those skills and cane manipulations, as described earlier in this chapter. In addition, the technique can be introduced after the student has learned to trail using the two-point-touch technique, which is described in the chapter that follows. The instructor choosing this last option has made the decision that because the student is working in an unfamiliar room, he should be using this cane skill, which was designed to be used in unfamiliar areas.

By the end of this unit, the student has gained enough self-confidence that he is ready to begin to explore unfamiliar environments. He does so first indoors and then outdoors, and he begins the process by learning to use the two-point-touch cane technique, which is described in detail in the next chapter.

Unit Two
ADVANCED INDOOR AND OUTDOOR ORIENTATION AND MOBILITY SKILLS

Chapters in Unit 1 covered environmental and spatial concepts and the specific skills that persons who are visually impaired need to begin traversing familiar indoor environments, as well as procedures for walking with a sighted guide and then for walking without assistance using self-protection techniques. The chapters in this section discuss how the O&M instructor teaches the student to use the cane in various familiar and unfamiliar indoor and outdoor settings.

In the exercise of long cane skills, it is more critical than ever that the cane be of the proper length because the incorrect length would render these skills not only ineffectual, but potentially dangerous. The advanced indoor orientation and cane skills described in Chapter 6 help the individual safely navigate through indoor settings, both familiar and unfamiliar. Therefore, it is imperative that the skills discussed in this and later chapters be taught exclusively by the O&M instructor.

Chapter 6 describes how to use the two-point-touch cane technique and its adaptations; presents detailed descriptions of self-familiarizations to hallways and buildings; and discusses the strengths and limitations of the cane techniques, sequencing and choosing environments for lessons, and direction taking and route patterns in indoor settings. Students receiving O&M instruction should be practicing these and other cane skills and demonstrate the ability to maintain their orientation throughout. They should also have begun to learn the techniques and procedures to reorient themselves to the environment if they become disoriented. Now they may be ready to begin the process out-doors.

In Chapter 7, procedures are described for teaching students to walk along sidewalks in a residential neighborhood and to detect curbs at street corners with the cane to avoid tripping off or falling into the street. Techniques for finding and using landmarks along the shorelines and using compass direc-tions and other outdoor clues and cues to remain oriented are also covered. Finally, ways of familiarizing oneself to street corners and city blocks are described.

Chapter 8 extends the area of instruction from the immediate environment of the student's home base to other blocks in the neighborhood. Procedures for crossing streets, the various configurations of streets, ways of recovering from veers when crossing streets, and the appropriate cane skills required to move through special environmental situations are described. Finally, techniques for familiarization to entire neighborhoods are included.

Chapter 9 deals with travel through various types of business districts, both small and large. Techniques for negotiating malls, rural areas, and special travel situations like alleys, gas stations, parking lots, and railroad crossings are explained. In addition, the chapter deals with how students learn to recog-nize their limitations and seek and accept assistance from passersby and how they can familiarize themselves to the inside and outside of stores.

6

Advanced Indoor Orientation and Mobility Skills

With the introduction of the basic two-point-touch cane technique, the student begins to learn to travel in unfamiliar or constantly changing indoor environments. Because her anxiety level may increase in these environments, she may fall back on previously learned skills and old habits, at least initially. The instructor takes this possibility into account and notes any hesitancy the student shows regarding travel through new and fearful areas and encourages the student with praise. Although the initial environment may, indeed, be familiar to the student, she becomes prepared to transfer these skills to a new, indoor travel area later on. The instructor reassures the student that he will be with her every step of the way as they begin to explore the new terrain together. The first step in this process is to learn the two-point-touch cane technique.

THE TWO-POINT-TOUCH CANE TECHNIQUE

The two-point-touch cane technique allows the student to probe the ground where she will place her foot next. In reality, the cane glides, slides, or pokes along the ground for an instant at two distinct points and provides the student with vital information on the level, texture, or composition of the surface and obstacles in her path. The student gathers this information as she walks, integrates it, and makes instantaneous judgments about her positioning along the route. The basic two-point-touch cane skill and its modifications become second nature to her over the course of her O&M program, so she concentrates on her orientation as she moves along. Therefore, the instructor ensures that the student has learned the proper cane skills indoors, where the environment is controllable and the terrain is flat and smooth, before venturing outside where the skills become more difficult to implement.

Basic Grasp and Cane Position

It is important for the student to hold the cane comfortably yet in a prescribed manner to receive appropriate feedback from the tip as it probes the terrain. The instructor will determine which procedure to teach, depending on the student's manual dexterity and cognitive and motor skills. The two basic procedures are the use of the fingertip method and that of the whole-hand method of grasping the cane.

THE FINGERTIP METHOD

- With her back squared off against a wall at the end of a long hallway, the student faces the instructor. The instructor holds the cane laterally as if he were shaking hands with it and places it in the student's dominant hand, which is positioned midway down the grip. The thumb rests on top of the grip, and the index finger is bent with its tip pressed firmly against the flat side of the grip. The third and fourth fingers are curled together and braced underneath the second finger, which rests immediately underneath the cane grip; they are all to be used as leverage.
- The instructor then inserts several fingers between the student's palm and the cane to create a space that will enable the student to pivot the cane separately from her palm. The grip rests along the knuckle between the fleshy part of the hand just beneath the thumb and the thumb itself (see Figure 6.1).
- The student's cane hand is held at her midline—at waist height or slightly above—with the arm extended forward and out from the body and the elbow slightly bent and braced against the student's rib cage. The student can also extend her arm completely away from her body if she wishes to.

The cane is held at midline to ensure the least amount of swing from side to side (arc width) from the center of the arc and ensures the maximum distance of the cane tip from both feet (see Figure 6.2). If the cane were held off to the dominant side of the body, the arc width would need to be wider to cover the entire width of the body, and the apex of the arc would be a shorter distance from the student's feet, which would cause the student to overstep the cane tip and, consequently, to trip off curbs or stairs.

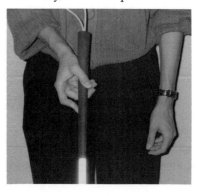

6.1 The fingertip grasp of the two-point-touch cane technique.

The hand is held at waist height or slightly higher, so the cane tip points at the least-acute angle to the ground, which ensures that the tip will remain close to the ground when the cane is swung from side to side because it naturally rises slightly off the ground during the walking phase of instruction, as described later. The preferred arc height at its apex, therefore, is one-half to two inches from the ground.

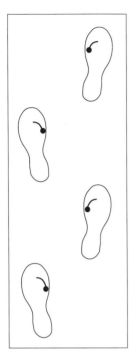

6.2 Proper cane tip touch-downs in relation to respective foot placements.

If the hand drops below the waist, the tip will probably rise higher off the ground during the arc swing. Thus, it will be harder for the student to determine whether she has felt a drop-off when the tip touches the ground. The student will discover that holding the cane hand below waist height will also cause it to poke into her groin when it contacts an object in her path. If she keeps the cane hand at the preferred height, however, it will rise and move away from her body when the cane contacts an object.

- The instructor faces the student and lightly grasps the wrist of the student's cane hand with one hand and the upper portion of the cane shaft with the other. He straddles the cane with the tip between his feet, so when the cane is swung, the tip will touch the inside portion of his feet exactly where he wishes the tip to touch down on either side of the student, creating the acceptable arc width of the cane. The ends of the arc width are slightly beyond the widest portion of the student's body to ensure complete coverage of the student's entire body width. The instructor thus ensures that when the cane is swung, the movements in the index finger and thumb are done properly until the student learns to feel the movements kinesthetically and can reproduce them herself. The hand, wrist, and arm remain stationary and in place throughout the cane swing (see Figure 6.3).

- The index finger is straightened to push the cane toward the nondominant side as the cane is "swung" to that side. As the finger relaxes and bends back into the initial position, the cane returns to the dominant side of the body. The fingertip remains on the cane and on the same spot on the cane as it pushes and relaxes.

- The cane is pushed or swung from side to side between the instructor's feet until the student relaxes her hand, wrist, and, hence, her cane swing. The student always begins swinging the cane to the dominant side from the nondominant side because she will use this procedure again when she learns to take her first step into a street to cross it. She will thus be in the habit of swinging it in this manner and will not have to learn a "new" procedure later.

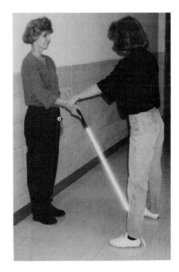

6.3 The instructor needs to ensure proper hand placement and arc width for the two-point-touch cane technique.

While the student is standing still, she keeps the tip on the ground as she swings the cane from side to side. The instructor notes the position of the student's hand and index finger throughout the swing to ensure that the wrist and arm do not move. When the instructor believes the student is learning to reproduce the proper finger movement, he lets go of the wrist and cane and allows the student to practice independently. When the proper arc width is attained, as evidenced by the cane tip gently touching his feet, he backs away from the student and observes the swing from a distance. He gives the student verbal feedback by telling her to "Swing the cane more to your right," or "More on the left," or "Less on your right side," and so forth.

THE WHOLE-HAND METHOD

• The student grasps the cane with the grip against the palm, the index finger pointing down against and along the flat side of the grip, and the fingers wrapped around the underside of the grip. She holds her hand laterally to the cane at midline and waist height and moves her wrist laterally side to side, from flexion to hyperextension to extension.

Using this grasp, the student must ensure that her wrist does not roll over as she swings the cane because the tip will then come off the ground higher than necessary and could cause the student to miss locating drop-offs with the cane, which could result in injury. Moreover, if the hand is kept at midline, when the wrist and hand move, it is difficult to monitor exactly where the tip is during all phases of the swing. The instructor follows the same basic procedure in teaching this grasp and swing as he did in teaching the fingertip method.

When teaching either method, the instructor takes care to note any postural abnormalities that may arise from the first attempt to hold and swing the cane in this manner: The student's dominant shoulder may become tight and lift up as her hand is held at midline and waist height (it can be massaged gently to relax and lower it); the head may be pointed down, up, or away from the midline as the student concentrates on feeling the movement; or the student's overall posture may generally suffer while she is learning the skill. In any event, the instructor begins to point out and correct these problems before they become learned behaviors.

Walking Forward while Swinging the Cane

STAYING IN STEP AND IN RHYTHM

After the student has demonstrated the ability to maintain the proper arm, hand, and wrist positions and has developed a constant arc width with either grip, she is then ready to move out and swing the cane while walking forward.

• The instructor explains how the cane is to be swung as the student walks. The student begins by swinging the cane to her dominant side and stepping forward with the foot of her nondominant side—for example, with the cane in her right hand, she swings the cane to the right and steps with her left foot. This is called staying "in step." As the student moves forward, the natural vertical displacement of her center of gravity will raise the cane tip slightly off the ground so that she will actually touch or gently glide the cane tip on either side of her body at the ends of the arc width. As the tip touches the ground, the heel of the foot that has swung forward will touch down. This is called staying "in rhythm" with the cane. It is important for the student not to try to "keep up with" her cane, but to swing the cane only as fast as she is walking; otherwise, she will appear to be pushing or "following" her cane tip. The student stays in step and in rhythm to ensure that the cane touches the ground where her foot will be placed next and thus detects obstacles or drop-offs; thus, the student can concentrate on her orientation to the environment.

• The student follows the instructor's voice down the hallway. The instructor makes such encouraging comments as, "Follow my voice; you're doing just fine," "Keep it up," "You're doing great," "You look real good," and "That's it." At first, the instructor stops the student if she gets out of step; later, he teaches her how to get back in step while moving—by touching the cane tip down twice on one side while in rhythm and then swinging it back to the other side. As the student moves forward, the instructor stays close enough for her to hear his verbal feedback and to keep her walking a straight line down the hallway (see Figure 6.4).

PROVIDING FEEDBACK TO THE STUDENT

If the student begins to veer, the instructor moves closer and asks her to follow his voice to get her back on track down the middle of the hallway. The instructor tries to avoid giving confusing feedback like "You're veering to the right" because it does not indicate whose right side he is referring to or whether he means that she should swing the cane more to the right or that she is actually swinging the cane too far to the right.

If the student's cane position falters during the movement forward, the instructor may model the skills while the student is in motion: He comes along the dominant side and slightly behind the student and molds one hand over the student's cane hand and rests his other hand lightly on the opposite shoulder. As they walk, the instructor actually swings the cane as he wishes it to be swung, with the student's arm, hand, and wrist in the correct positions; with the proper arc width and height; and in step and in rhythm. As the student relaxes her grasp of the cane and begins to swing her free

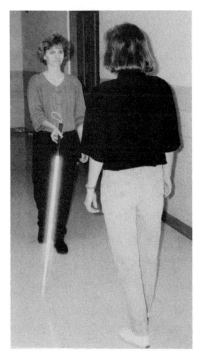

6.4 The student learns to stay in step and in rhythm using the two-point-touch cane technique.

arm more naturally and seems to perform the technique more appropriately, the instructor relaxes his grasp of the student and eventually lets go of her.

INSTRUCTOR'S POSITION WHILE MONITORING THE CANE SKILLS

As the student moves forward independently, the instructor observes her cane skills from various positions. First, from the front, he observes the position of her arm, hand, wrist, and cane; the width and height of the arc; and her general posture. Second, from the side, he observes the student's arm extension and where the cane tip touches down in relation to the next foot placement: whether it touches an imaginary line where the ball of the foot will touch next or if the foot touches down either in front of (*overstepping*) or behind (*understepping*) the line where the cane tip will be placed next. From the rear, the instructor notes the arc width, the position of the student's arm, and the student's ability to stay in step and in rhythm. Later, adjustments in the location of the cane grasp on the grip (either up or down), the arm extension (either closer in to or farther out from the body), the length of the stride (shorter or longer), and the length of the cane may have to be made to compensate for any consistent disparity.

Turning and Trailing

EXECUTING TURNS

Once the student has demonstrated consistent cane skills while walking I–routes along the hallway, she is ready to walk more complicated routes while maintaining the proper touch technique throughout the turns. Turning is done as follows:

- As the student turns, she swings the cane toward the turn and steps with her opposite foot in the direction of the turn.
- Just before the student comes to the intersecting hallway, the instructor tells her when to begin to make the turn so she has enough time to be in position to turn down the new corridor gradually.
- Later, the student determines for herself when to begin to turn by slowing down when she thinks she has come to the corridor and listening for the opening.
- If the student gets out of step during the turn, the instructor models the technique in the same way he did earlier.

TRAILING A WALL

When the student demonstrates a consistent cane technique as she walks in open spaces, she is ready to learn to use the two-point-touch technique to trail along a wall. The instructor first chooses a wall that is devoid of obstacles and recessed areas, so the student may learn the skill. As the student becomes proficient in trailing, the instructor introduces walls with obstacles, doorways, recessed areas, and protruding objects. The student learns to trail a wall using the following procedure:

- The student stands parallel to and nearly at shoulder-touching distance from a wall along her nondominant side.
- With the cane in her dominant hand, she rests the cane tip against the baseboard of the wall.

- She takes her first step forward by simultaneously swinging the cane tip to the dominant side and stepping forward with the foot of her nondominant side, so she is in step and in rhythm.
- She proceeds to walk along the wall line using the two-point-touch technique, but lightly touches the baseboard of the wall each time she swings the cane to the wall line.

The student maintains a constant distance from the wall as she trails along it. She always touches the baseboard at the same point along the arc width, that is, at the widest portion of the arc along her nondominant side. If she drifts away from the wall, she swings the cane farther to that side, and if she drifts closer to the wall, she touches it nearer at her midline. The instructor provides verbal feedback as the student trails along the wall, and the student makes the necessary corrections accordingly. The instructor follows the same procedural sequence described in Chapter 5 for diagonal cane skills.

The student always keeps the cane in the dominant hand when using the two-point-touch technique, even when trailing the wall on the dominant side (see Figure 6.5):

- With the wall on the dominant side, the student rests the cane tip up against the baseboard.
- As she swings the cane to the nondominant side, she simultaneously steps forward with the foot of her dominant side and continues along in step and in rhythm.

Modifications

Occasionally the situation may warrant modifications of the two-point-touch cane technique. The flexibility of these modifications, which are described in detail next, enables the student to travel in all types of situations. For instance, the student may wish to use the constant-contact technique when traveling on tile floors to avoid drawing attention to her cane because of the loud tapping sounds. She may wish to use the touch-and-slide technique to locate curbs or stairs or the touch-and-drag procedure to find the railing from the top of a staircase. And she may wish to use the three-point-touch technique to

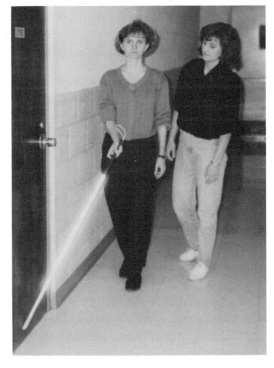

6.5 The student locates a door while trailing a wall and using the two-point-touch cane technique.

locate an intersecting sidewalk after making an errant street crossing. Some students, especially those who have multiple impairments, may prefer to use a particular modified technique all of the time.

In any event, these procedures are derivatives of the basic two-point-touch cane technique and are learned when the need arises. That is, they are not introduced and practiced in any one unit, but are taught when the instructor deems it appropriate to do so. They are all described here for the reader's convenience.

CONSTANT-CONTACT CANE TECHNIQUE

The constant-contact technique is used when the student is first learning the two-point-touch technique in a stationary posture and when the student wishes to keep the cane tip on the floor or ground. It ensures the earliest possible detection of a drop-off and does not draw attention to the student by the sounds of the cane tappings on the floor or ground. The technique is helpful for persons with multiple impairments and others who have difficulty detecting changes in the terrain.

Essentially, the technique consists of the student's keeping the cane tip on the ground while swinging it back and forth and keeping in step with the cane as it reaches the ends of the arc width. The technique has its drawbacks, however. The cane tip is likely to stick in cracks in the sidewalk and in other rough areas. Students with weak hand grasps will find it difficult to use this technique over long periods because it requires sustained muscle control and some dexterity. Furthermore, students may have difficulty staying in step without the tactile and auditory cues of the cane tip tapping the ground.

TOUCH-AND-SLIDE CANE TECHNIQUE

The touch-and-slide cane technique is used when the student wishes to make as much contact with the ground as possible but the terrain is not smooth enough to allow the tip to stay constantly on the ground. It is also used to locate drop-offs and to determine changes in the terrain, such as from a sidewalk to compacted mud or gravel. When compacted wet leaves or a solid layer of snow or ice covers the sidewalk, the student can use the technique to "poke" down into the covering to feel for the sidewalk to avoid veering off the intended walking surface. Finally, some students use the technique to differentiate between dry spots and puddles along their paths of travel. In the touch-and-slide technique, the student uses the two-point-touch technique, but allows the tip to slide forward along the ground several inches at each touching down of the cane. She appears to be poking the cane along the ground as she walks.

TOUCH-AND-DRAG CANE TECHNIQUE

The touch-and-drag technique is used to trail a shoreline outdoors or to remain parallel to a drop-off while walking along it. For instance, if the student wishes to locate a railing at the top of a wide staircase, she positions herself parallel to the edge of the steps and uses the touch-and-drag technique along the edge to maintain a safe and constant distance from the drop-off; she walks until she finds the side or end of the steps, where she can locate the railing.

In this technique, the student uses the two-point-touch technique trailing procedure, but after the tip touches the ground to the side opposite the trailing surface, she drags it back along the ground to the trailing surface. Thus, the cane touches down along one side only. For example, if the shoreline is on the left, the student begins with the tip up against the shoreline and swings the cane off the ground to the right side and touches the cane tip down. She then drags the cane along the ground back to the shoreline and repeats the procedure. Each time she swings the cane, she still maintains her hand at midline, and her cane and feet are continually in step and in rhythm.

THREE-POINT-TOUCH CANE TECHNIQUE

The three-point-touch cane technique is used to detect objects located off to the student's side and above the level on which she is walking. It requires more coordination than do the other techniques and may, therefore, require the instructor to model the technique as an essential teaching approach. The student generally stands in the street parallel to the curb along which she will be trailing or at the base of a stairway.

- With the cane tip placed against the shoreline, the student steps forward with the foot closest to the shoreline and swings the cane away from the shoreline and touches the tip down (Point 1) at the widest point of the arc on that side to keep in step; as the tip touches down, the forward heel strikes the ground to keep in rhythm.
- As the rear foot begins to come forward, the cane swings back to the shoreline and the tip touches the base of the shoreline (Point 2) at midstance and before the heel strikes down.
- Just as that heel strikes down, the cane tip is elevated over the edge of the shoreline and simultaneously touches down (Point 3) several inches on top of and into it to locate landmarks or intersecting walkways or sidewalks.
- From the top of the shoreline, the cane swings back to the initial point (Point 1), and the procedure is repeated until the object on top of the shoreline (such as a handrail, landmark, or preferred sidewalk) is found.

The instructor models the technique by standing along the dominant side and holding onto the student's cane hand with one hand and to her far shoulder with the other hand. He then helps the student swing the cane while ensuring that her hand and the cane are in the correct position and that she is in step and in rhythm. The technique is also used to locate doorways along building storefronts because it enables the student to hear and feel the differences between the bases of the building and the glass or metal doors. The student touches the cane twice along the building line: at Point 2 she touches the base of the building, and at Point 3 she touches just above the base. Since the technique is used in more advanced travel situations, it is generally introduced later in the student's O&M program.

ONE DOWN AND ONE UP-OVER

One down and one up-over is used for the same reasons as is the three-point-touch technique, but many students find it easier to accomplish. It does not, however, provide the student with information about the exact location of the shoreline. Basically, it is the same as the two-point-touch technique, only the cane tip extends over and onto the shoreline as it touches down on that side and does not touch the edge of the shoreline. Therefore, the student may have difficulty maintaining a consistent distance from the shoreline to detect openings to stores, walkways, and driveways, and this difficulty may be mistaken for simple veering away from the shoreline. This technique can be implemented over and onto grass at the same foot level as the student; over a curb from the lower street level; or along a storefront, "one down and one up": The cane tip touches down on the ground on one side, and up and gently against the storefront on the other side.

Stairs

ASCENDING STAIRS

After the student has become familiar with the two-point-touch technique, she may then be ready to travel on different floors of a building. To do so, she must learn to travel up and down stairs independently using her cane. Because the floors are unfamiliar to her, it is recommended that she first learn the two-point-touch technique before she attempts to negotiate stairs independently. Since the student may not be able to rely on railings at all times, she first learns to negotiate the stairs without the use of railings. (As was mentioned in Chapter 3, some railings end prematurely or wind around the staircase, and some staircases do not have railings.) It is more difficult to teach the student how to traverse stairs without handrails if she first learns to do so with handrails. Therefore, after she demonstrates the ability to negotiate stairs without railings, she then learns how to locate and use railings.

However, it should be noted that some students, such as those who are overweight, who have balance problems, or who cannot feel their feet beneath them, must always use railings because of their physical impairments. In any event, the instructor determines how the student will traverse the stairs with or without railings and explains the entire procedure with the student's back against a wall and away from the stairs.

The instructor first explains and then shows the student the following procedure:

- The student approaches the stair riser using the two-point-touch technique, plants the cane tip up against the riser, switches over to the pencil-grasp diagonal cane position, and walks up to her cane so the tip is between her feet and her toes are pointing forward and touching the riser.
- To determine where along the steps she is located, the student then runs her vertically held cane along the riser to her right with the cane in her right hand, and to her left with the cane in her left hand. She judges the distances to the railing on either side to position herself at an equal distance between them.
- With the cane in the pencil-grasp diagonal cane position and held on the shaft just below the grip and at her midline, the student checks the height of the first stair step by lifting the cane tip off the ground and up to the edge of the step.
- She then checks the depth of the step by running the cane tip from the edge of the

step to the riser of the second step. Generally, she can infer that the rest of the steps on this flight are of equal height and depth.

- With the cane tip held vertically and in the pencil grasp, the student repositions the tip between her feet and on the floor. She then counts to the third step by lightly touching the cane tip on the edge of each stair step.

- The student locks her elbow so her arm is held straight out in front of her, parallel to the ground with the hand and cane at midline. The cane tip is barely touching the lip of the third step.

- The student leans forward and proceeds to walk up the flight of steps, one foot on each step. The cane tip lightly bounces off the lip of each step until it reaches the landing, where it floats into open space. The student takes care to ensure that the tip does not lag behind and get between her feet when she is using the pencil grasp (see Figure 6.6).

- The student walks up the remaining two steps and repositions the cane into the two-point-touch technique and locates the next flight of steps. The procedure is repeated until both the student and instructor feel confident that the skill is learned. Once the procedure is learned and demonstrated satisfactorily, the student does not need to check the height and depth of the first step on each flight, especially if the staircase is familiar to her.

During this exercise, the instructor positions himself behind the student, holding on to the railing with one hand and wrapping his other hand around the student's shoulder—making physical contact only if the student loses her balance. As the student becomes more adept with the skill, the instructor remains on the lower landing (or several flights below) while the student negotiates the stairs independently. At first, the student is positioned in the center of the staircase to avoid bumping into the handrails if she should veer. Over time, she may wish to position herself along the right side to climb with the flow of traffic.

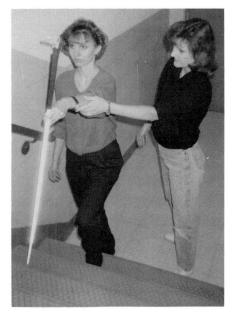

- A modification of the pencil grasp is for the student to hold the cane at a diagonal to her body while using the pencil grasp for protection against unexpected objects or obstacles on the stairs.

- As a second alternate grasp, the student can use the thumb grasp of the diagonal cane technique, holding the cane at a slight diagonal from her dominant side to her nondominant side. The student avoids following the cane up

6.6 The student ascends stairs while using the pencil grasp of the diagonal cane technique.

the stairs because both her cane hand and the tip are off to her sides, and this circumstance could cause her to veer.

DESCENDING STAIRS

As in the stair-ascension procedure, the instructor explains the entire procedure to the student with the latter's back to a wall and away from the stair's edge. It is especially important that the student does not stand over the descending staircase for long periods because her knees can lock with anxiety and fear, causing her to lose her balance or faint. The instructor uses a reassuring voice and has the student come to his voice to approach the stairs. He positions himself on the staircase, one or two steps below the landing, holds on to the railing for balance and support, and ensures that the student finds the edge of the landing with her cane tip. The following procedure is used:

- The student approaches the edge of the landing using either the constant-contact or the touch-and-slide technique. When the cane tip drops off the edge, the student locks it up against the stair edge and cautiously approaches the edge with her feet on either side of the tip and her toes resting slightly over the edge.
- She then holds the cane vertically and runs it along the riser of the first step down in either direction, first in one hand and then in the other, to determine her position on the landing. She takes care not to lean too far in either direction when searching for the side of the stairs. She carefully sidesteps to center herself on the landing.
- With the cane held on the grip in the pencil-grasp position, the student raises the tip to the landing edge and back down to the first step to determine the height of the steps.
- She then runs the tip along that step from the riser to the edge to determine the depth.
- To ensure that her feet are pointed directly ahead, she then runs the shaft just above the tip along the toe of each shoe. She places the cane in the right hand to trace along the right foot, and in the left hand to trace along the left foot. She repositions her feet until each foot is equidistant from the center of the toe to the stair edge on the side of it.
- She then grasps the cane using the index-finger grasp of the diagonal cane technique: She holds the cane at the top end of the grip for maximum extension, bracing her hand against the lateral side of her thigh for support and a constant point of reference.
- As the student stands erect, she points the cane down the stairs with the tip slightly off the edge of the first or second stair step from the landing.
- She leans back slightly as she begins her descent, one foot on each step, maintaining the cane and hand position throughout; the tip does not touch any step until it locates the landing.
- She walks down the remaining two steps as the cane tip glides along the landing and walks away from the stairs using the two-point-touch technique. She finds

the next landing edge and repeats the procedure until both she and the instructor are confident of the consistency of her technique.

The instructor walks down the stairs backward as the student descends. He holds on to the railing and observes the student, giving her encouragement as she negotiates the steps and ensuring her safety throughout. The instructor is careful not to obstruct the student during the descent, and moves out of the way when the student reaches the landing (see Figure 6.7).

In the procedures just described, the student is positioned in the center of the staircase for both the ascent and the descent. This position is necessary at first to ensure that she does not bump into the railings and lose her balance if she should veer. Later, the student may prefer to be close to the right side to take the flow of traffic into consideration.

LOCATING AND USING A HANDRAIL

After the student becomes adept at negotiating stairs with no railings, the instructor shows her how to locate and use a handrail, when one is present and one hand is free to hold on to it:

• The student locates the stair edge or riser using the two-point-touch technique and turns to the side to put it parallel to her.
• She then uses either the touch-and-drag technique (for descending) or the two- or three-point-touch trailing technique (for ascending) until she finds the side of the stairs or the railing.
• While facing parallel to the stairs, she positions her cane vertically against the side wall or railing and puts the cane into the hand closest to the steps. She runs the cane along the wall until the shaft makes contact with the railing.
• She slides her cane hand down the shaft until it contacts the railing and grasps it with the other hand for stability and support.
• She turns and faces the steps, placing the cane in either the pencil-grasp position for ascending or the index finger grasp for descending.
• She negotiates the stairs using the cane skills described earlier for ascension or descension, but she lets her other hand slide along the railing and in front of her body. When this hand locates the end of the railing, she completes the procedure, relying solely on her cane to detect the landing.

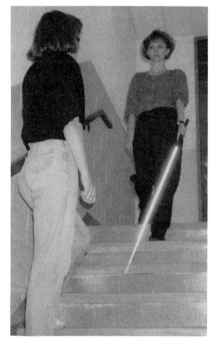

6.7 The student descends stairs while using the index finger grasp of the diagonal cane technique.

Familiarization with Hallways and Buildings

Many students now have all the prerequisite skills to learn how to become familiar with an unfamiliar floor of a building or an entire building. Floor and building familiarizations are extensions of the basic room-familiarization procedure, but on a larger scale. The student demonstrated earlier that she is capable of orienting herself to an unfamiliar room. She now has the mobility skills necessary to protect herself from obstacles or hazards that are commonly found in most buildings and can travel from one floor in a building to the next using the stairs. This orientation skill is first learned in concert with the instructor; then with only a minimal amount of assistance from him; and, finally, with no assistance. The student learns one floor at a time until she is oriented to an entire building. She is then given the opportunity in a series of lessons to orient herself to a different building.

During this mini-unit, the student has ample opportunity to practice and solidify her cane skills, refine her indoor orientation skills, and develop the self-confidence necessary to begin outdoor travel. At the end of the O&M program, she may have gained enough confidence in her skills to familiarize herself to most indoor travel areas. Therefore, the instructor takes care not to "teach to" a particular floor or building, but teaches a process that can be applied to any floor or building. This philosophical approach differentiates a mobility aide or technician from the mobility specialist. It is up to the latter to distinguish between the learning of an environment for the particular environment's sake and ensuring the transferability of learned O&M skills to any other travel environment.

FAMILIARIZATION WITH THE FLOOR OF A BUILDING

The process is the same as the room-familiarization process and will not be redescribed here. It is, however, easier to accomplish in theory than in practice. The instructor guides the student through the process, taking each hallway as a separate entity. One hallway is treated like a room and is learned thoroughly before another hallway is added. The same thoroughness is applied to every hallway. The difficulty is to help the student determine which course of action to take at critical junctures. That is, since few hallways are surrounded by four walls, there may be at least one intersecting corridor, and the student must learn how to treat it. The diagrams in Figure 6.8 may serve as an example.

In this illustration the floor is H-shaped, with two parallel hallways connected by an intersecting, perpendicular hallway. The student enters the floor from any one of the four exit doors at the ends of the parallel hallways and uses that door as her reference point, or home base, for the next several lessons. She "discovers" the size, shape, and contents of the floor through the self-familiarization process detailed in Chapter 5. Therefore, only the differences and nuances will be described next:

- After the student explores the door and door wall, she selects a wall to trail and branches out along the corridor.
- She trails along that wall until she reaches another wall in front of her or an "out-

side" corner (one that turns away from her) that would indicate an intersection. She always returns to her home base upon locating an area that requires a change in direction.

- If she locates an outside corner, she returns to her home base and then trails along the opposite wall, estimating the same distance and looking for another outside corner that would indicate an intersecting corridor in both directions, creating a "+" intersection. If she does not find a corresponding outside corner, she surmises that the intersection dead ends at this hallway, creating a T-intersection.
- She returns to the original outside corner by trailing the opposite wall around and back along that wall until she locates the opposite outside corner and crosses over to complete the route back to the home base.
- If she locates an inside corner, she simply renegotiates the area and branches out along a new wall until she completes a circumference of the hallway.
- She then runs routes to and from objects along the walls in the hallway until she becomes comfortable with their locations in relation to each other. By this time, she is able to identify landmarks and name the walls using the landmarks or using compass directions (or both).
- She begins a series of routes in open spaces in the hallway to reconfirm its shape.
- She now is ready to enter the opening and explore a new hallway in the manner just outlined.

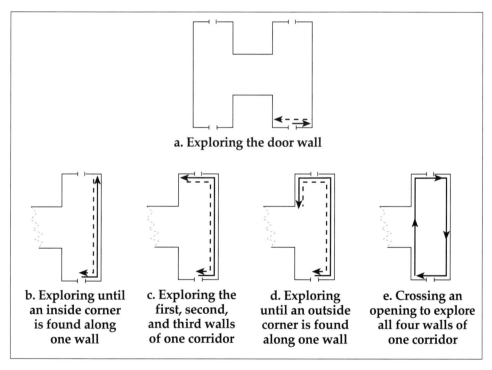

a. Exploring the door wall

| b. Exploring until an inside corner is found along one wall | c. Exploring the first, second, and third walls of one corridor | d. Exploring until an outside corner is found along one wall | e. Crossing an opening to explore all four walls of one corridor |

6.8 Floor familiarization: One hallway on an H-shaped floor.

- She adds one corridor after another in a similar manner.
- After she has run numerous routes in each of the corridors, mixing trailing and walking in open spaces and locating objects in one corridor and then in another, she may be ready to explore other areas on the floor, if appropriate. She has already noted any exit doors or other doors with glass windows. Glass windows generally signify that an area is open to the public. She therefore selects a door with such windows (or an exit door) and enters the new area, seeks assistance to determine if she has any interest in exploring it, and explores it if she does. If there are no such areas, she is ready to explore a different floor of the building.

FAMILIARIZATION WITH AN ENTIRE BUILDING

The student treats each floor of a building in the manner just described, learning one floor at a time and maintaining compass directions consistently throughout the mini-unit on each floor. She learns stairwells as she readies herself to go to the next floor. When a new floor is learned, she walks routes to the previous floor or floors and the newly learned floor; for example, from the water fountain in the elevator hallway of the first floor to the women's rest room on the third floor.

Consistencies among floors are inferred and verified during the process. That is, the student expects to find plumbing fixtures (rest rooms and drinking fountains) in the same locations on each floor, stairwells and elevators in similar locales throughout the building, and a consistent numbering system throughout the building. Thus, what she has learned on one floor should be transferable to every other floor, with some exceptions at times. That is, after she learns one unfamiliar floor, the student is already somewhat familiar with all the other floors. Understanding this concept makes the process less threatening and, for many students, more motivating to learn.

CONSIDERATIONS FOR EFFECTIVE TEACHING

Suggestions for Teaching the Fingertip Grasp

One easy method for teaching the fingertip grasp of the two-point-touch technique is to ask the student to point toward the ground with the dominant hand. The instructor adjusts the student's fingers so the index finger is bent slightly and the fingers are curled one under the other. He then places the cane in the student's hand so the index finger is along the flat side of the grip; the thumb is resting on the top of the grip; and the grip is resting on the second, third, and fourth fingers.

Limitations of the Two-Point-Touch Cane Technique

Because the cane is swung from side to side and, sometimes, onto different surfaces and surface levels in each procedure, it is inevitable that the student will miss objects as she moves along. The most vulnerable areas are those immediately surrounding the body, primarily above, below, and to each side of the hand and cane and around the head, chest, and knees. In addition, the cane tip may simply not detect a drop-off, or the student may misinterpret the information she is receiving from the cane. The student learns these limitations and uses caution when traveling, especially in unfamiliar areas. Using the upper hand and forearm procedure when trailing along a new wall helps to protect the upper body from protruding objects and unexpected open doors. A slower stride allows for a quicker reaction time to unexpected events and obstacles. Some electronic travel aids (see Chapter 10) are early-warning detection systems that enable the traveler to identify and locate oncoming hazards that would normally not be detected in the usual cane procedures. In any event, the student takes the necessary precautionary measures when traveling with a long cane to lessen the possibility of injury.

Strengths of the Two-Point-Touch Cane Technique

Despite the limitations just described, the two-point-touch cane technique and its modifications are the most reliable techniques for detecting and sensing the environment for nonvisual locomotion and travel. When the student combines them with educated judgments about the environment, she can travel safely and efficiently through nearly any travel environment and situation. As was mentioned earlier, the two-point-touch technique enables the student to concentrate on her orientation to the environment without worrying about her next foot placement or whether she will trip off the sidewalk and into the street. This knowledge greatly reduces her fear of travel and increases the student's belief in her ability to avoid becoming disoriented or lost.

Sequence of Lessons and the Instructor's Position

Lessons continue to build on one another; additional skills are constantly introduced and the responsibility for remaining oriented in and moving independently through environments shifts to the student. The familiarization lessons present the opportunity to shift this burden. At the beginning of the mini-unit, the instructor provides the instruction and a great deal of feedback. He moves throughout the route patterns, giving information about things the student would not notice: subtleties of the cane hand and wrist movements, staying in step and in rhythm, postural inconsistencies, reasons for disorientation, and the like. As the student takes command over her movement, the instructor becomes more of an observer and provides feedback and encouragement after the route or lesson.

Overlearning the Two-Point-Touch Technique

The initial lessons in this technique are tedious for both the student and the instructor. Instructors can break up the monotony of the initial lessons by concentrating on one or two facets of the technique, reviewing previously learned skills for a brief period, and then returning to drill on the technique. Many fine-motor skills are integrated and learned and are added to gross-motor movements. The swinging of the cane with the index finger is first learned in a stationary posture. To integrate this fine-motor skill, the student overlearns it before progressing to other aspects of the technique. The instructor encourages this overlearning by first determining the parameters of the acceptable behaviors. For instance, he decides that he will accept the finger movement as "learned" when the student demonstrates the ability to swing or move the cane from side to side between her feet without banging each foot during the swing. He sets the arbitrary limit that if the student lightly touches each foot 10 consecutive times, she has learned the skill. But to ensure overlearning, he sets the limit a little higher, say, to 15 consecutive times for each foot. Once the student demonstrates proficiency and consistency, the skill may be thought to be overlearned.

As the instructor adds other skills to the process, he expects that the student's proficiency in the overlearned skills will drop off initially. Theoretically, skills should diminish only to the acceptable "learned" parameters. As the student begins to move into the environment, her cane skills may diminish further, but after the skills are integrated, they may return to acceptable levels. (The concept of overlearning, as well as the dissipation of skills, applies to all motor skills. See Chapter 1 for a more detailed discussion of overlearning.) Furthermore, the instructor should expect skills to diminish whenever new environments are introduced, when unusual situations arise, or when new units of instruction are begun. It is imperative, therefore, that skills be overlearned and reinforced constantly and consistently.

One way the instructor can remind the student to use the proper skill without calling attention to the deficit, especially between lessons, is to devise a mutually agreed-upon code word or number that will trigger a reminder of when to initiate the proper form or procedure. For example, the two might agree that whenever the student hears the instructor call out the number "five," she knows that the instructor has observed her being out of step and she should correct it immediately. To reinforce the skills of all his students, the instructor can use this same code. If he walks down the halls of the agency or school calling out the code, he may note one student realigning her hand at midline, another checking that she is in step, and a third standing more erect.

Students learn that motor skills are to be performed outside the mobility class, as well as during class time; are best developed in a real-life setting; and must become second nature to them. Therefore, the instructor informs other teachers, parents or relatives, and even other students of the various motor-skill areas that require practice and asks them to reinforce the proper behaviors so the student will practice her skills whenever walking to and from various classes or locales.

Selection of an Environment

The initial lessons in the two-point-touch technique can be given in the same indoor training areas used for previously learned skills. As the student learns to familiarize herself to unfamiliar indoor areas, additional buildings must be found so she can learn to transfer the skills. It is not necessary to find high-rise buildings for this process, but buildings with several floors, consistent floor plans, intersecting hallways, and a small amount of pedestrian traffic would be excellent training facilities. Examples of acceptable buildings include churches; schools; libraries; factories; post offices; and state, county, and local government offices. It may be necessary to obtain permission to work in some buildings, so care should be taken to do so before beginning the lessons.

Orientation and the Questioning Process

As the student moves more independently through the environment, she will inevitably become disoriented. How the instructor questions the student will determine, in large part, whether the student will become an independent traveler and the level of confidence each will have in the student's travel abilities. Thus, giving the student the answers will only get her through a particular situation; it will not prepare her to find her own answers after instruction is completed. The questioning process is one of the most difficult aspects of teaching O&M to persons with visual impairments.

The instructor first determines if the student has the skills and experience needed to determine independently where she is after she becomes disoriented. If she does not, the instructor does not expect her to reorient herself. Verbally questioning the student at the time of the apparent confusion helps the student begin to consider the questions she will be silently asking herself later: "Why do you believe something is wrong?" "When was the last time you knew you were on the right track?" "Did anything unusual happen to you when you were walking after that time?" "Which way should you be facing?" These and other questions do not elicit a one-word response or give away the answer.

After the student determines where she is, she must then decide what she did to become disoriented. "Why do you think this happened?" "What should you have been attending to while you walked along?" "What can you do the next time this situation arises?" These and other questions put the responsibility squarely on the student's shoulders.

Finally, the student must get back on track and complete her route to the intended destination. "What direction are you facing?" "What direction should you be facing?" "What landmark should be coming up?" "What part of the route pattern are you on?" "Where will you go to get back on track?" "How will you know when you get there?" The questioning process can then be paired with the instructor's guiding the student back to the point of confusion either physically, by using the sighted guide technique, or mentally, by drawing a map of the situation on the student's hand or back. In later lessons, the latter technique is preferable because it is more convenient and because it allows the student to learn to make corrections from the current location, rather than having to go back to the point of confusion and start from there. Eventually, the map written on the hand or back is replaced by the mental map that the student creates and uses independently.

Route Patterns for Practice

Route patterns follow the same sequence as in earlier lessons, from simple I-routes to Z-routes, in which turns are practiced and various objects are located in the halls.

As the student begins the familiarization process, route patterns are incorporated into the lessons to learn the floors of buildings and the buildings themselves. The instructor should expect the student to maintain the proper skills, especially when the environment is unfamiliar.

Working with Persons Who Have Low Vision

Some students with residual vision may need to learn the two-point-touch cane technique, especially if they have only a small amount of vision or restricted fields of view. As with the diagonal cane technique, these students may need to learn to rely on the cane and use their remaining vision for orientation. Many instructors have made excellent use of blindfolds or low vision simulators to introduce and practice a skill. They may take the simulators-occluders off the student after she has learned the skill so the cane skill can be paired with the visual input. When learning to become oriented to a building, the student learns the spatial layout and how to find landmarks visually while using the cane for protection from obstacles and drop-offs.

Working with Children

Depending on their ages, many children can learn from the sequence of instruction outlined in this chapter. The fingertip method of grasping the cane may be ineffectual for young children who have not yet developed fine-motor hand skills, but they may still benefit from the whole-hand method. Some children may need to be taught in or near their home environments for the lessons to be truly meaningful. Furthermore, lessons may need to be shorter in duration or divided into sublessons; for example, one-third of the lesson may be a review of the previous lesson; one-third may be new material; and the last third may be something totally unrelated, such as a playground or gym activity. For other children, instructors may create games to teach the skills. Hide and Seek, Treasure Hunt, Follow the Leader, and Simon Says are some games for younger children that are perfect for learning cane techniques and even orientation to rooms, floors, and buildings.

By the end of this process, the student should have had ample opportunity to refine her cane skills and develop a solid foundation for more advanced O&M skills. After the development of and much practice in indoor skills, many students may be ready to build on this foundation and apply these skills to outdoor travel.

7

Basic Outdoor Orientation and Mobility Skills

The student may now be ready to begin traveling outdoors. This chapter deals with how the instructor selects an area for instruction that will provide the student with a range of experiences in initial outdoor travel. Outdoor travel entails complicated situations involving complex decision-making strategies by both the student and the instructor. If the student is technically but not emotionally ready for outdoor travel, the instructor must find ways to ease the student outdoors. Some instructors introduce students to "campus" travel in an agency or school complex—one that is familiar to the students and the least threatening. If students are being taught in their home areas, the initial instruction may take place in their driveways, along the sidewalk that is nearest to their yards, or on the grounds of their churches, for example.

Good instructor-student rapport and constant reassurances are the keys to overcoming many students' fears of outdoor travel. The instructor introduces the series of units of instruction described in this and the next several chapters by attempting to control the variables as much as possible while allowing the student to begin to make his own judgments and to take responsibility for his own actions. The student begins to learn to walk along sidewalks, to explore them for usable landmarks, and to maintain his own orientation. As the student's skills increase, the burden of responsibility shifts from the instructor to the student, as it did for indoor travel.

CHOOSING THE SETTING

Whether the instructor decides to begin the outdoor travel process on a confined campus or in a residential neighborhood, she must consider a number of variables. She must assess the proximity of the locale to the student's home if she is teaching itinerantly or to the school or agency in which she and the student are based.

Although she may find an "ideal" setting for instruction, it may be too far away to allow for enough actual instruction time. The instructor looks for an overall environment from which to teach the entire residential unit. Ideally, areas for initial lessons should have well-defined sidewalks and curbs and identifiable landmarks, and pedestrian and vehicular traffic should be at a minimum so the student can concentrate on his cane and orientation skills. Later lessons, as described in subsequent chapters, incorporate more heavily traveled areas and more challenging sidewalks and street patterns and lead into small- or medium-size business districts. In sum, the instructor notes the parameters of the prospective teaching environment, that is, the boundaries of the surrounding streets, and the potential driving distances and times from the student's home or the agency or school.

Assessing the "Quality" of the Setting

The instructor must also assess the quality of the teaching environment to answer the following questions: Does the setting provide appropriate experiences that are controllable? Are some sections of the area less frequently traveled by pedestrians and vehicular traffic and other sections more heavily traveled? Are there definable landmarks? Is there a discernable pattern to the layout of the area? And, is the area large enough to be sectioned off to provide for a transfer of skills before a new unit of instruction is started?

To answer these questions, it is helpful for the instructor to walk the proposed area using a long cane, if her student is a cane traveler, to "feel" the terrain as the student will eventually do. What appears easy to detect or note when viewed visually may be difficult to discern when using a cane. In some respects, beginning outdoor travel in a residential area is more difficult than in any other outdoor travel area because the student does not yet possess advanced orientation skills as part of his repertoire. The instructor notes this problem when preparing for introductory outdoor training.

In the basic outdoor lessons, the instructor looks for clearly defined sidewalks, if available, so the student need not fear the prospect of directly encountering passing vehicles. Such sidewalks have easily discernable shorelines on either side, and detectable curbs at either end. One sidewalk along a particular street intersects with another, and a third, and so on, so a city block is formed with sidewalks along each of its sides. The sidewalks are smooth enough for the easy use of the two-point-touch technique. The shorelines have definable edges with intersecting driveways and walkways.

Street "Furniture"

Along the shorelines one may find numerous pieces of street "furniture" that can be used as potential landmarks. Street furniture includes objects like fences and walls, shrubbery, street and traffic signs, mail boxes, and fire hydrants or plugs. Each area of the country has its own types of street furniture, and, depending upon the student's needs, the instructor will emphasize learning how to locate and identify furniture native to a particular area or the types of furniture that can be located in different areas of the country. It is important for the instructor to be aware of the names used for various objects in various parts of the country. For instance, walkways in some areas of the country are called sidewalks in other areas. The strip of grass between the sidewalk and curb is a parkway, grassy area, or tree lawn, depending on where one lives.

Sometimes, further distinctions are made between similar objects simply for the sake of clarity. That is, sidewalks and walkways are differentiated from each other because they lead to two distinctly different places. Walkways are the cement pathways perpendicular to the sidewalk. They lead from the house to the sidewalk and often to the curb. Sidewalks, on the other hand, are the cement areas that parallel the street and lead from one street corner to another. Therefore, the instructor may wish to avoid confusion by referring to either or both as a sidewalk, especially at critical times, such as when she is questioning the student during periods of disorientation. Since sidewalks have two shorelines, one is termed the *inside* shoreline because it is closer to the house, and the other is designated the *outside* shoreline because it is closer to the street or curb. Sides of a walkway are not differentiated.

Some types of street furniture are more likely to be found along one shoreline than the other. For example, gates and walls are usually found along the inside shoreline of a sidewalk, whereas street signs and fire hydrants are usually found along the outside shoreline. By learning these consistencies, the student begins to understand the outdoor environment and is able to make more educated judgments about his exact location if he becomes disoriented.

Progression of Lessons

Outdoor lessons progress in the same manner as do indoor lessons. The student first learns the cane skills necessary to negotiate sidewalk travel. He builds on his knowledge of the sidewalk from walking down the middle of it to exploring the shorelines. He builds on his knowledge of the block from traveling along its sides to explore its corners discretely. Finally, he mixes walking down the middle of the sidewalks and trailing the shorelines to locate specific landmarks and objectives. During these lessons, the instructor goes from assisting to observing as the student assumes more responsibility for his actions. At first, the instructor stays close to the student as the student walks down the sidewalk, but as the student gains proficiency, the instructor backs away from him and observes his cane skills from all sides and provides adequate and timely feedback. Once the student understands the corner-familiarization procedure, described later in this chapter, the instructor merely observes the accuracy of the procedure and the subsequent routes to and from designated landmarks.

SIDEWALK TRAVEL

During the initial lessons, the instructor emphasizes the mechanics of walking along a sidewalk. The student's cane skills usually drop off somewhat at this time because sidewalks, however smooth they may appear to be, are considerably rougher than are indoor tile floors. At this stage of the mini-unit, orientation skills are deemphasized until the cane skills are refined.

- The student begins at one end of the sidewalk with his back to a street and walks from one end to the other while following the instructor's voice to maintain a straight line of travel; following the instructor's voice also helps to alleviate his fear of walking inadvertently into the street. As the student nears the far corner, the instructor reminds him to switch from the basic two-point-touch technique to the touch-and-slide technique to ensure that he will locate the impending drop-down, or curb. The student slows his pace to detect the curb without stepping off the sidewalk and into the street. At this point, the instructor has stepped into the street and positions herself at the curb edge to ensure that the student does, indeed, detect the curb with his cane. If the student does not detect the curb, the instructor does not allow him to trip off the curb into the street.
- The instructor and student repeat this procedure numerous times up and down the sidewalk until the instructor no longer feels the need to be in front of the student. The instructor observes the student from behind and along his side as he walks down the middle of the sidewalk and detects the curb edges consistently.

Straight-Line Travel

The importance of straight-line travel should not be underestimated. The straighter the line of travel, the easier the travel skills become and the more likely the student will use his skills after the O&M program has concluded. Because the constant sticking of the cane into the shorelines can be disconcerting and can sour the student on traveling outdoors, the problem should be corrected as quickly as possible. Likewise, since veering may cause him to lose his walking rhythm and to sway too much from side to side, which can also cause pinballing, it is important for the student to continue to move forward and to use the elbow of the cane arm as a shock absorber to lift the cane tip up slightly and over the sidewalk crack and back onto the pavement without losing his rhythm and the intended line of travel.

Therefore, the instructor finds ways to help the student ensure a straight line of travel:

- If the student pinballs along the shorelines even when following the instructor's voice, the instructor can walk directly behind him and physically guide his shoulders to make the slight body realignments necessary to correct his position, similar to what was done indoors in the hallways. The instructor knows that the student may not necessarily be veering in as much as the "passageway" has, in fact, narrowed, when compared to traveling indoors. Thus, the student may narrow his arc width slightly to compensate for a narrower passageway than was found indoors.
- It may be helpful for the student to "visualize" the sidewalk area as a narrow hallway with imaginary walls where the shorelines are located. He tries to walk as he had done indoors with ever-so-slight readjustments in his direction after his cane contacts the shoreline. He tries not to allow the cane to contact the same shoreline more than twice consecutively.

- The student may also find it helpful to imagine "seeing" himself walking in front of himself and to follow the image down the center of the sidewalk, as he did earlier with the instructor's voice. This videating technique alleviates some the anxiety of travel. Since the student is always following a "friend" and thus "sees" the unfamiliar area before he actually walks into it, the new territory cannot truly be unfamiliar to him.

Whatever the reasons for the pinballing or cane stickings into the shorelines, the eventual outcome should be a consistently straight line of travel from one curb to another. The instructor must find a way for the student to reach this outcome as quickly as possible. By allowing the student to pinball or constantly contact a shoreline, the instructor limits the student's eventual travel abilities and ensures that additional problems will arise later. All travel should be done in the middle or to one side of a sidewalk, as directed by the flow of traffic, with as little contact with the shoreline as possible.

Shorelining

The purpose of shorelining is simply to find a landmark or a particular destination or to reconfirm an intended line of direction. The student should limit his shorelining because shorelines lead to driveways, wide parking lots, and alleys, all of which are potentially hazardous and disorienting. The potential of veering into these areas should be avoided unless they are intentionally being sought out. However, some students, especially those with multiple impairments, who would become disoriented without having a shoreline to rely on, may find it necessary to follow a shoreline when traveling. In these instances, shorelining should be done on the correct side, as directed by the flow of traffic.

To shoreline, the student follows one or more of these procedures:

- With the shoreline parallel to him on his nondominant side and his closest foot nearly up against it, the student swings his cane from the shoreline to the dominant side and steps forward with the foot of his nondominant side.
- He continues to swing his cane and stays in step and in rhythm as he walks along the sidewalk.
- He swings his cane back onto the shoreline with the proper arc width on that side, so the tip touches down several inches over the shoreline's edge and onto the grass.

The instructor ensures that the student maintains the proper hand position and grasp of the cane throughout the exercise and models the procedure if the student has difficulty manipulating the cane. The student practices shorelining on one side of his body before he learns to do so on the other side, until he exhibits consistency. If the student has difficulty using the basic two-point-touch trailing procedure, the instructor shows him one of these two alternate methods:

- The student uses the touch-and-drag or three-point-touch technique along the shoreline, as described in Chapter 6. Either requires a refined cane technique and may result in even more cane stickings than does the two-point-touch technique.

- The student uses the two-point-touch technique but keeps one foot on the shoreline as he walks, maintaining a constant distance and hence a straight line of travel. With this procedure, the student may step into uneven shoreline areas and soil his shoes.

If the student veers away from the shoreline, he can turn his head and "look" toward it, as he did the wall indoors, which should keep him close enough to the shoreline. Veering away from the shoreline should be avoided because the cane will eventually contact the sidewalk pavement, which easily can be mistaken for a walkway or driveway. The student could then miscount the number of driveways and walkways, which would lead him to the wrong destination.

The instructor mixes practice in walking in the center of the sidewalk and shorelining to locate objects along the side of the block. After walking numerous routes along all sides of the block, and eventually interjecting compass directions and street names into the routes, the student is ready to learn to find and use landmarks at the corners of the block, which is preparatory to becoming familiar with an entire block and, eventually, an entire residential neighborhood.

STREET-CORNER FAMILIARIZATIONS

The student will eventually walk through residential neighborhoods from street to street and hence from the corner of one street to the corner of another. In most instances, his orientation will be centered on the concept of a street "corner," rather than the concept of a street "block." That is, he is more likely to need to know at which corner of an intersection he is, rather than at which corner of a block. Therefore, the instructor should be careful how she describes this critical information to the student. Although blocks have four corners that are identifiable through compass directions, these corners have different designations compared to the other corners of their respective intersections. For example, because the northwest corner of any block is also the southeast corner of that intersection, the designation coincides with its diagonally opposite counterpart. This concept is difficult for many students to distinguish; as a consequence, confusion can be avoided by simply introducing the designation in relation to the intersection, as in the exercise that follows.

The exercise has two basic components. First, the student determines on which corner of an intersection he is standing. Second, he determines the landmarks he should use to identify that corner in the future.

Determining the Exact Corner of an Intersection

To determine the corner of the intersection, the student must first know the direction of one compass point. If he does not, the instructor points it out before beginning the procedure. For the sake of this discussion, north will be in front of the student, as will the perpendicular street, and the parallel street will be to his right.

- The student stands on the corner and faces the perpendicular street with his feet just in front of the curb's edge; the instructor stands either directly in front of the student and in the street facing him or directly behind him.

- The student determines one compass direction and the positions of the two streets in relation to his body.
- The instructor and student engage in a dialogue similar to this one:
- *Instructor:* "You are facing north and the perpendicular street is in front of you. The perpendicular street is, therefore, what compass direction to you?"
- *Student:* "North of me."
- *Instructor:* "Then, what direction are you to it?"
- *Student:* "I am south of it."
- *Instructor:* "Good; remember that compass direction for later. You are on the south side of the perpendicular street. Now, where is the parallel street?"
- *Student:* "To my right."
- *Instructor:* "Good. What compass direction is to your right?"
- *Student:* "East is to my right side."
- *Instructor:* "If east is to your right, then the parallel street is what direction to you?"
- *Student:* "It is east of me."
- *Instructor:* "Then, you are what compass direction to it?"
- *Student:* "I am west of it."
- *Instructor:* "Excellent. You are, therefore, on the west side of the parallel street. Now let's put all of this together. You are south of the perpendicular street and west of the parallel street. Therefore, you are on the southwest corner of this intersection."

The instructor and student practice this exercise facing either street and at each of the corners of the intersection until the student can determine the corner himself each and every time.

To aid in this exercise, the instructor may develop a tactile map of the intersection and use it while she explains the procedure during the process, itself. A model of the intersection, although more cumbersome than a map, may also help the student understand the concepts involved. The model can even show miniature cars and how they travel on the streets and through the intersection. Eventually, the student moves from using the model or map to picturing the intersection mentally to determine the corner designations. The map or model should be presented in the same mental plane in which the student visualizes. That is, if the student visualizes in an aerial plane, then the map should be held flat in his hands or on a table; if the student visualizes on a frontal plane, then the map should be held directly in front of him, as if it were up against a wall. Likewise, if the instructor chooses to draw the map on the student's back or hand, she should take into consideration which plane is the best representation for his student.

Finding Landmarks at Street Corners and Midblock

Now the student may be ready to find the usable landmarks at the initial corner. This procedure enables him to develop a consistent and reliable method for doing so. While facing a perpendicular street, he always starts with the inside shoreline and moves away from the parallel street when starting to explore. He always returns to a curb edge when approaching the perpendicular street. And he always completes the procedure by returning to the curb edge of the original perpendicular street. In this manner, he will explore every point along the street corner, is less likely to miss an object, and will remain oriented throughout the many turns in the procedure.

At first, the student will locate all objects at a corner and note their relative locations. As was mentioned earlier, these objects are common to the neighborhood, but their location relative to the corner and to each other will determine whether they are suitable to be chosen as landmarks. Possible objects include fire hydrants, street signs, street-light poles and guy wires, walls, fences, shrubbery, and mailboxes. As the student learns more about each of the corners along the block, he will designate one object or configuration of objects as the landmark for that corner. He will further limit his landmark determinations as he learns more about the corners of other intersections while he explores the entire neighborhood.

He begins to explore the corner by following this procedure:

- Facing the perpendicular street and standing near the curb edge, the student locates the inside shoreline and trails it away from the curb edge as it winds around the corner and becomes the outside shoreline of the newly designated parallel street. He exaggerates the shorelining cane technique by swinging his cane well into the tree lawn, so he can explore all the objects that are set back away from the shoreline and note their order to each other along the shoreline from the corner.
- After a short distance, he crosses over to the inside shoreline, and trails back to the corner, crossing the intersecting sidewalk and locating the curb edge of the originally designated parallel street, which now is his new perpendicular street. He learns to recognize that he is no longer facing the original perpendicular street and compass direction. He further notes any objects he has come into contact with and their locations to each other.
- He then repeats the process: He follows the inside shoreline as it winds around to become the outside shoreline, crosses over to the inside shoreline, and trails it back to the curb edge at the corner. He has now returned to the original curb edge and is facing the original perpendicular street and compass direction.
- He checks with his cane to determine if there is a grassy area between the intersecting sidewalks along the curb edge and then explores this area either by shorelining along the sidewalk edge or by using an exaggerated touch-and-drag technique along the curb edge and well onto the grassy area, or a combination of both (see Figure 7.1).

REMEMBERING ONE LANDMARK PER CORNER

One common aid to memorizing the numerous objects is a tape recorder. The student records each object as he comes upon it, and its relative location on the corner. Later, he can compare corners and determine which objects to designate as landmarks. He can save this information on tape for later reference and keep the recorder with him while walking through the neighborhood, in case he ever becomes disoriented.

After noting the combination of common objects and their locations by identifying the particular shoreline and the particular street, the student notes which combination will be used initially as the designated landmark. He follows the same procedure at the next corner of the block and then walks routes to and from objects or landmarks at each of the four corners until he is successfully walking routes throughout the block from landmark to landmark. For example, he goes from the fire hydrant on the outside shoreline of one corner to the stone wall along the inside corner of another corner. One corner may not actually have anything that can be designated a landmark, but the absence of any objects may be unique to a particular corner and thus may be, in and of itself, the landmark. After exploring all four corners of the block, the student tries to limit each corner to one identifiable landmark, if possible.

After the student has thoroughly learned to identify and use landmarks at the corners of a block, he is then ready to explore and locate landmarks midblock. Once again, these landmarks can be common objects, or they may be subtle changes in the terrain, such as slopes to the side that may designate driveways or slopes in front of him that may designate oncoming hills.

NEGOTIATING SLOPES

The student learns to negotiate slopes in front of him by adjusting his cane grasp, either up or down on the grip, and his arm extension. For uphill slopes, he will choke down on the cane toward the base of the grip and shorten his arm extension; whereas for downhill slopes, he will choke up on his cane and extend it out as far from his body as possible. In either instance, he is attempting to create the same cane extension and distance from his body as if he were on level ground. Lateral slopes are more difficult to negotiate because he must keep the slope consistently lateral to him as he walks across it in a straight line. Although one foot will be higher than the other, he must be careful not to walk down the slope and possibly into a street or up the slope and into a driveway.

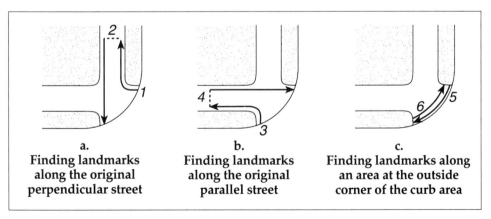

a.
Finding landmarks along the original perpendicular street

b.
Finding landmarks along the original parallel street

c.
Finding landmarks along an area at the outside corner of the curb area

Figure 7.1 Finding landmarks at street corners: The street-corner familiarization.

CONSIDERATIONS FOR EFFECTIVE TEACHING

Orientation Clues

The student initially relies on tactile clues as landmarks for maintaining his orientation. As he gains experience traveling in the residential area, he learns to attend to other clues as well. Compass directions play an important role, especially when combined with other pieces of information, such as street names, traffic patterns, and the flow of traffic. For example, the primary streets in a residential area may run north-south and have names that have particular meaning to the neighborhood. These names may reflect the theme of a particular subdivision; for instance, the Turtle Creek subdivision may have street names like Turtle Creek Court, Tortoise Run, and Painted Turtle Cove. Other neighborhoods may have streets named for the U.S. presidents or trees or flowers. Secondary streets in this example run east-west and are numbered, First Street, Second Street, and so on; the street numbers may get higher as they go from north to south in a neighborhood or city.

The student is generally interested in listening for traffic sounds to determine the differences among primary, secondary, and tertiary streets. Primary streets are wide and heavily traveled by large vehicles and usually have stoplights. Secondary streets are not so wide; have less traffic, especially large vehicles; and are often controlled by stop signs. Tertiary streets are narrow, have sporadic traffic, and do not always have traffic controls. One-way streets have cars traveling in the same direction on both sides of the street, which distinguishes them auditorily from the traditional two-way streets. Therefore, if the student notices a large number of vehicles on a particular parallel street, he may conclude that it is a primary street. It should hence be running north-south. To determine exactly which way is which, he may need some additional pieces of information—about the sun, the terrain, and the traffic.

THE SUN

For the student to use the sun for orientation purposes, he must know the time of day and remind himself of the time of year. For instance, in the northern hemisphere, the sun generally remains in the southern portion of the sky and, therefore, rises in the southeast, is overhead in the south during midday, and sets in the southwest. During the summer, it is more traditionally overhead, rising in the east and setting in the west. Obviously, the student can use the sun only when it is visible—not when clouds cover it or when the student is in a shaded spot. Therefore, the sun is not as reliable as are other clues.

By noting the position of the sun and identifying a shoreline as inside or outside, the student can interpret which side of a street he is on and which direction he is facing (or wishes to be facing). Going back to the foregoing example, the student determines that it is nine o'clock in the morning and the sun is to his right side; thus, east is to his right. He then locates a shoreline with his cane, identifies whether it is an inside or outside shoreline, aligns to it to confirm the position of the sidewalk and parallel street (to his left, in this case), reconfirms the position of the sun, and is able to determine that he is on the east side of a primary street and facing north.

THE TERRAIN

Changes in terrain are subtle indicators that warrant the student's attention. Sudden slopes, sidewalk endings, and gravel areas where pavement should be all cue the student to attend to and analyze what is happening.

THE TRAFFIC

Listening to the traffic may further indicate that the student no longer is on the desired primary street. Noting that the cars are all going in the same direction may also indicate exactly which street the student has wandered onto and help him determine which way he should go to get back on track. The most difficult thing the student has to accept is the possibility that he has erred; he then has to determine what is happening around him. He learns to listen for environmental sound clues, and then to explore for landmarks that will aid in his reorientation. Once reoriented, he must determine a course of action to get himself back to his route so he can continue on to reach his destination. The advanced traveler will be able to devise an alternate route to get back on track, and it should be the most direct course of travel.

During this introductory mini-unit to outdoor travel, the student has not yet developed the repertoire of skills to accomplish the reorienting process just outlined. However, as situations occur during the lessons, the instructor introduces the student to a particular step in the process. Therefore, she devises enough lessons and routes that inevitably will produce situations in which such moments will present themselves.

Knowing When to Move on

When the student exhibits a consistent cane technique, whether for sidewalk travel or shorelining, he may then be ready to add another cane skill. As he displays an understanding of basic orientation skills—locating and using landmarks—he may be ready to add his knowledge of compass directions, traffic, streets and their patterns, and the sun for more advanced orientation cues. Generally, when clues become cues, and the latter become the recognition of the current location, then the student has begun to integrate and use higher-level orientation skills. Tactile skills must eventually give way to auditory and other sensory skills.

Developing Meaningful Lessons

Adding one skill to another merely splinters the learning process. If the lessons can become meaningful to the student, whether a child or an adult, then he is more apt to integrate and use the skills when the O&M program ends. The instructor can aid in this process by establishing a home base (a designated house in the neighborhood, if not the student's own home) to use as the starting point of each lesson. The student learns to identify this house along the shoreline of the sidewalk and pretends that he is learning his own neighborhood. Every sidewalk, every street corner, and every street now have meaning to him. The houses he locates in subsequent lessons will be the homes of his "relatives" and "friends." Discussions between lessons will inevitably lead to more information about the student's home area if it is different from the teaching area, and provide the instructor with vital pieces of data from which to develop meaningful lessons. As the lessons become meaningful to the student, he may become motivated to learn the skills necessary to travel in more advanced environments.

The Traveler with Low Vision

Whether or not the student is a cane user, he will need to understand the layout and configurations of a residential area. Many instructors ask their students to draw low vision maps of the area. By using a blank piece of white or off-white paper and a black felt-tip pen, the student can draw the layout of the area and place traffic signs, street names, and appropriate destinations on the map. This activity focuses the student on those aspects of the area that are critical to him: shapes of blocks, visual landmarks (the colors of certain houses; particular trees, shrubs, and fences; and the like), the locations of house numbers and street-name signs, and other signage, if warranted. Many students with low vision need to learn to use monocular telescopes to help them read addresses and street signs and must learn the correct angles for reading the signs in relation to the lighting conditions.

These basic skills are fundamental for the student to learn to branch out farther into the residential neighborhood. He may now be ready to explore different city blocks and learn how to become familiar with entire neighborhoods. But to do so, he must first learn to cross streets, as described in the next chapter.

8

Intermediate Outdoor Orientation and Mobility Skills

The student may now be ready for a series of lessons on crossing streets safely and consistently. When students learn these skills, they are able to travel through and explore different city blocks within residential areas and refine their long cane and orientation skills. Initial street-crossing lessons are conducted in a quiet section of a residential area, so the instructor controls as much as possible situations that could compromise the student's ability to gain the skills and confidence necessary for successful travel. As the student's skills and confidence develop, lessons progress to different types of travel situations, such as intersections that are offset or have dead ends and more heavily traveled areas.

CROSSING STREETS WITH NO TRAFFIC

Crossing a Perpendicular Street

Initial street-crossing lessons are conducted in the absence of traffic, so both the student and the instructor can concentrate on the basic mechanics of the procedures with no fear of approaching vehicles. As the student learns later, street crossings are easier to negotiate in the presence of traffic because of the auditory cues from cars and the person's own ability to discriminate and localize traffic sounds. However, crossing streets with traffic requires a degree of self-confidence that the student cannot develop before she learns the mechanics of the street crossing itself. The basic street-crossing procedure is accomplished first at two- and four-way stop intersections, where the perpendicular street traffic must stop.

In the first several street crossings, the instructor simply guides the student across the street so the student can get a "feel" for the crossing. In the next several crossings, the student tells the instructor when it is safe to cross, making this determination by the absence of traffic sounds. The crossings are made using the sighted guide technique. Over time, the student learns to discriminate traffic sounds several blocks away, which do not pose a hazard to the crossing, from those within close proximity. To begin the crossing, using her cane, the student approaches the corner using the touch-and-slide technique until she feels her cane tip slide off the curb edge and then locks the tip up against the edge (as she has done while descending stairs).

REALIGNING TO THE SHORELINE

If the student contacts a shoreline as she approaches the corner, she may have lost her direct alignment with the opposite corner. Therefore, she must turn around and walk back away from the corner, realign herself to the inside shoreline, and reapproach the corner. If she does not do so, she may wind up facing away from her intended line of travel with no indication that she has done so until she attempts the street crossing.

To realign using the shoreline, the student faces in the direction of the corner, stands parallel to the inside shoreline, places her foot up against the shoreline, and sweeps the cane along the sidewalk and back to the shoreline. She attempts to feel the shoreline's edge with her cane tip in relation to her body position so she can determine that it is just off the shoulder and closer to the inside shoreline and that she is, as a result, parallel to it. This is a procedure similar to the one used indoors against a wall line: If the shoreline feels as if it is farther off to the side of her shoulder, the student interprets this to mean she is facing away from the shoreline; if the shoreline feels as if it is more toward the midline, then she may be facing it. She wishes to be parallel to it, that is, neither facing into it nor facing away from it. Once she is realigned, she reapproaches the corner until her cane tip drops off the edge of the curb.

- The student inches her way forward, taking care not to turn her body until her feet are several inches from the curb's edge; she plants her feet so the dominant foot is slightly forward of her nondominant one, and her weight shifts slightly forward onto the dominant foot. She takes extreme care not to move her feet until she executes the crossing, since even a small amount of movement can cause her to face away from her intended line of travel.
- To determine whether there is an obstacle in the street immediately in front of her intended path of travel or if there is a deep gutter or puddle of water, the student switches at this point to the diagonal cane position, using the index finger grasp with the cane tip against the curb's edge and in the street and her cane hand at midline.
- She sweeps her cane tip along the ground in a semicircular motion from the nondominant side to the dominant side, while keeping her hand at the midline throughout the sweep. She returns her cane tip to midline and drags the tip back to the curb's edge to check for obstacles within the arc of the imaginary semicircle, which covers the area of the first footfall.
- Finding no obstacles or deep gutters, the student places the cane in the "ready-to-cross" position: The tip is placed out of the street and up against the non-

dominant foot; the cane is grasped using the index finger grasp of the diagonal cane technique, palm outward with the arm extended from the body and at the midline.

- The student practices this part of the procedure numerous times until the instructor sees that her skills are consistent and she performs them without hesitation.
- In the ready-to-cross position, the student swings her cane just off the curb's edge and into the street to the dominant side where that foot will eventually step down. Simultaneously, she steps off the curb with her nondominant foot. (This is the same procedure used to begin swinging the cane in the two-point-touch technique learned indoors.) The instructor ensures that the first footstep is directly forward, because it is critical to the student's alignment as she crosses the street. The instructor stands in the street facing the student and provides feedback regarding the position of the cane tip and the first foot placement. Some instructors prefer their students to "flag" or swing their canes three times before stepping off the curb to signal motorists of their intention to step into the street.
- The student practices this critical first step and cane placement numerous times without allowing the dominant foot to leave the curb's edge. The instructor ensures that the cane tip does not come off the curb more than several inches during this phase to avoid potential injury to an oncoming pedestrian.

After practicing the step-off, the student is now ready for the actual crossing:

- The instructor asks the student to come to his voice as she uses the procedure just described. After the first step-off, the student is now in step to swing the cane using the two-point-touch technique. She walks quickly across the street until she locates the curb's edge at the corner on the opposite side. By moving quickly, she ensures a straight line of travel and avoids being in the street longer than is necessary. She follows the instructor's voice to the approaching curb's edge, plants the cane tip up against the edge, and walks up to the tip so her feet are on either side of it, as she did to approach ascending stairs indoors. The instructor steps behind the student until the student steps up onto the curb at the corner.
- The student clears a path in front of her by sweeping the cane once along the sidewalk of the street corner from the nondominant to the dominant side. Simultaneously, she steps up onto the street corner with her nondominant foot as her cane tip reaches the dominant side. She completes the crossing by continuing to walk forward away from the curb's edge while staying in step and in rhythm. Some instructors prefer their students to sweep their canes in a spiral pattern before stepping up onto the corner to detect possible objects in their path or features of the terrain.
- The student crosses and recrosses the same street from corner to corner until she performs the procedure with refinement and speed.

INSTRUCTOR'S POSITION

As the student gains proficiency, the instructor provides fewer and fewer auditory cues. He moves from being in front of the student and having the student follow his voice across the street to being next to and slightly behind the student before and during the crossing. As the student is readying to cross the street, the instructor stands slightly behind and away from the parallel traffic sounds, or just on the inside shoreline. This position keeps him from interfering with the sounds of the parallel traffic, allows him to monitor the traffic from all the streets simultaneously as it enters the intersection, and to allow him to intervene physically, if necessary, if the student starts to cross at the wrong time. As the student initiates the crossing, the instructor moves behind the student and slightly away from the parallel cars so the student is between him and the parallel traffic. In this manner, the instructor stays close to his student if the need to intervene arises, yet he does not block the sounds of the parallel traffic, which can be useful in readjusting one's alignment while making the street crossing. I–shaped routes are then negotiated, incorporating numerous street crossings along the selected parallel street.

ALIGNING TACTILELY TO A SHORELINE AND A CURB
If the student has difficulty approaching the corner to face directly across the perpendicular street, she may position herself next to or with one foot on the inside shoreline and run her cane along the curb's edge to ensure that the edge is perpendicular to her, as she did when descending stairs. She then positions her toes over the curb's edge and checks them with her cane to determine that her feet are facing squarely across the perpendicular street. This practice does not entirely ensure that the student is facing appropriately in that it is difficult to determine that the curb's edge is not, in fact, curving around her. The student may square off to a curved curb and be actually facing into or away from the intersection.

Crossing the Parallel Street
After consistently crossing the perpendicular streets in the neighborhood, the student is now ready to learn to cross the street parallel to her initial alignment. On doing so, she will be able to "box" an intersection by crossing to all four corners to learn what landmarks she will use to become familiar with the immediate area.

There are two ways to cross the parallel street: first, by crossing the perpendicular street and then the parallel street and, second, by crossing the parallel street without first crossing the perpendicular street. The first procedure is easier than the second in that it involves fewer turns and, hence, less chance of misalignment.

BY CROSSING THE PERPENDICULAR STREET FIRST
• On completing the street crossing, the student steps up onto the street corner and takes a few steps forward to place herself on the path of the crosswalk of the parallel street (or the crosswalk area if none exists).
• She then turns 90 degrees in the direction of the parallel street to face it. Using the touch-and-slide technique, she reapproaches the corner to the curb's edge of what was once the parallel street and has now become her perpendicular street.

The instructor takes care to help the student learn to make sharp 90-degree turns. If the student makes a sharp and accurate turn, she will be facing directly across the new perpendicular street in the crosswalk area. If she does not make accurate and consistent turns, it may be necessary to create a mini-unit on turning at the street corner or, in some instances, indoors, where the environmental conditions are more favorable to practice turning. (For more information on developing lessons on turns, see Considerations for Effective Teaching in this chapter.)

BY CROSSING THE PARALLEL STREET FIRST

• On approaching the perpendicular street, the student turns around 180 degrees to face away from the perpendicular street, takes a few steps forward to place herself in alignment with the crosswalk of the parallel street, and turns 90 degrees toward the parallel street.
• She then approaches the new perpendicular street until her cane tip drops off the edge of the curb and follows the basic street-crossing procedure from this point on.

The student uses the first procedure to "box" an intersection. That is, she crosses the streets in a counterclockwise or clockwise fashion until all four corners have been reached in either circular direction. She thus creates an imaginary box that incorporates all four corners of the intersection as the respective corners of the box, with the center of the box being the intersection itself.

Creating a Tactile Model of the Intersection

For many students, especially those who were born with a visual impairment, the instructor may wish to create a tactile model of the intersection to help them conceptualize it at the intersection or at the agency or school. The model may incorporate four city blocks, with the imaginary "fifth block" connecting each of the four corners of the intersection. The instructor cuts four rectangles out of plywood, form board, or artist's canvas to represent the blocks and then cements them on a piece of hardboard to form an intersection. He cements thin strips of sandpaper onto the blocks to create the sidewalks and crosswalks. He then places thumbtacks into the blocks at the respective corners of one intersection and connects them with rubber bands to create the "fifth" block.

CROSSING STREETS WITH TRAFFIC

After the student learns to cross the streets with no traffic sounds, she may then be ready to learn to use the traffic as an aid for alignment and as a determinant of the proper time to initiate the crossing. In reality, there have been stop signs controlling the traffic at one of the streets at the intersection, but the traffic has not yet been a factor. As the student moves into more advanced areas of the residential area, she begins to encounter streets with a greater frequency of traffic. She cannot depend upon a time when traffic will be absent long enough to make the crossing safely. Depending on the residential area, the student's ability to use the traffic will depend upon the type of traffic controls available. If there are no traffic lights, for example, the instructor will introduce them to the student in a more advanced travel environment later. Because traffic-light-controlled intersections require traffic to be completely stopped or completely going, they are easier to negotiate than are stop-sign intersections. Although traffic is supposed to stop and go alternately at stop-sign-controlled intersections, in reality traffic at best slows down before going through the intersection.

Types of Intersections

TWO-WAY STOP-SIGN INTERSECTIONS
• If the stop signs are on the parallel street, the student gets into the ready position and listens for the traffic on the parallel street to come to a complete stop. As one vehicle surges forward and the student determines by listening that the vehicle is not turning, she initiates the street crossing using the traffic as a buffer between her and the perpendicular cars.
• If the stop signs are on the perpendicular street, the student gets into the ready position and listens for the traffic on the perpendicular street to come to a complete stop. She starts crossing immediately thereafter, once she has determined that there is no parallel traffic. If there is parallel traffic, she crosses as one vehicle reaches its nearest corner of the intersection and after she determines that it has not slowed down to initiate a turn. This is a more advanced crossing technique used by very competent and confident students. For other travelers, it may be more appropriate to wait for an absence of all traffic at these intersections.

FOUR-WAY STOP-SIGN INTERSECTIONS
• In the ready position, the student listens for the surge of a vehicle in the parallel street after determining that it will not be turning.
• The student then initiates the crossing while listening closely to the perpendicular vehicles to ensure they are not yet moving.

THREE-WAY STOP-SIGN INTERSECTIONS
• When a one-way and a two-way street intersect, the student assumes the ready position and listens for the surge of a vehicle in the parallel street after determining that it will not be turning.
• The student then initiates the crossing while paying close attention to the perpendicular cars.

INTERSECTIONS WITH TRAFFIC LIGHTS
• In the ready position, the student begins crossing after the parallel traffic begins to surge through the intersection and after she determines that the first surging car is not turning right on the red light.
• At first, students may learn to cross such intersections using traffic sounds as an indicator of when it is safe to cross. Later on, students are shown how to locate crosswalk buttons and to use them to aid in their street crossings.

Intersections with Crosswalk Push Buttons

Students learn that although crosswalk push buttons are usually found on telephone poles in close proximity to the crosswalks, the buttons are sometimes found on especially designed poles that are self-contained units. Sometimes the poles are not so close to the crosswalk areas as they should or need to be and may be difficult to locate. Since there is usually one button to push for crossing a particular street, a pole may contain two buttons. These buttons may be located on the pole facing the street to be crossed, facing away from the street to be crossed, or facing parallel to the intended street crossing; printed arrows typically indicate to the seeing pedestrian which button is for which street crossing. Therefore, the nonvisual traveler may have to push a button and listen to the traffic to determine when the traffic is stopping and on which street. It may take several attempts to discover the traffic pattern and the correct button to push. The student should push the button several times to ensure that the signal is engaged.

In general, in all the instances of crossing just described, the student learns to make the easiest possible crossing—when two one-way streets intersect—taking the traffic controls, the flow and pattern of traffic, and "live" and "dead" lanes into consideration. In this type of crossing, the student crosses when the traffic on the parallel street flows in the same direction in which she is traveling and when the perpendicular street traffic must stop at the crosswalk directly in front of her. Because the lanes of perpendicular traffic are all "dead" lanes in that no traffic is or can be moving in them as she crosses, she must attend primarily to the sounds of the traffic next to her on the parallel street. At an intersection of two streets that are two-way streets, however, the student must attend to the traffic sounds of both streets and take into consideration both dead and live lanes of traffic. "Live" lanes of traffic are those in which traffic is moving or has the potential to be moving.

Auditory Alignment Using Traffic Sounds

The student also attends to the exact location of the traffic as it moves through or idles at the intersection. In the example presented in Figure 8.1, the student attempts to cross at a plus-sign intersection where two streets intersect. She listens to parallel traffic on her left and notes that if she is facing correctly, the idling cars are located at seven o'clock and at eleven o'clock to her. Cars on the perpendicular street are idling at nine o'clock and at one o'clock. Furthermore, moving cars on the parallel street are heard laterally coming from behind to midline at its farthest point and moving laterally in front of her to her midline at its farthest point; that traffic sound will never cross her midline. Likewise, the perpendicular traffic will stay in front of her as it passes by from right to left or from left to right and will never get behind her. The student points directly at the sounds of the moving or idling traffic to ensure accurate sound localization. The instructor helps the student localize this moving traffic by pairing the sounds with the position of the student's cane either parallel or perpendicular to her. As the instructor positions the cane up against the student and parallel to the particular traffic sounds being identified, the student runs her hands along the cane as she listens to the traffic sounds.

Sound localization and discrimination may be difficult if the sounds are masked or shadowed by other sounds or objects. Sound shadows are created by objects between the student and the attending source of the sound. For instance, sounds are shadowed or muffled if the student is standing next to a traffic-control box or a mailbox that blocks the traffic sounds as she listens for the parallel cars. If a jackhammer is masking or overriding the sounds of the traffic, the student may have to go to another intersection to cross safely.

In any event, the student determines that the conditions are exactly right for crossing the desired street. Therefore, she must patiently wait for these conditions to occur and ignore any distractions. The student learns not to accept the word that it is safe to cross from well-intentioned passersby. Unless those individuals

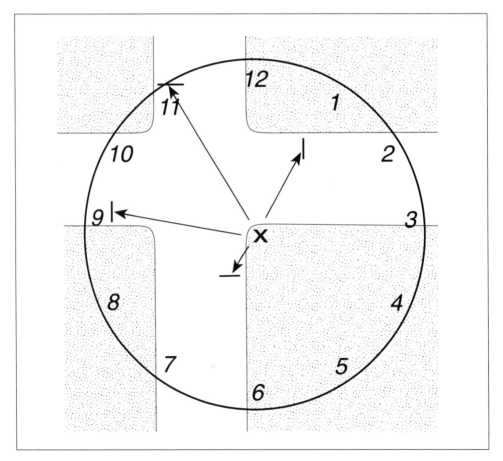

Figure 8.1 Auditory alignment using the positions on a clock face.

are willing to escort the student using the sighted guide technique, the student should cross only when she herself determines that the timing and conditions are right.

CROSSING AT OTHER INTERSECTIONS

At a T–(or dead-end) intersection, the student should follow these procedures:
• When crossing from a corner to traverse across the street forming the crossbar of the T–intersection, the student initiates the crossing when the parallel car begins its turn into the intersection. It is safer to cross when that car is going away from her or when she steps into a dead lane of traffic. After crossing, the student looks for a landmark to use to recross the street back to that corner at some later time.
• When crossing from the top of the T to a corner, the student must find a location to align safely for the crossing. She either listens for the traffic sounds and estimates the location of the opposite corner or finds a landmark to use.

Even advanced travelers may find crossing at T–intersections a formidable task. The uncertainty of the crossing and of having audible traffic sounds on which to rely makes this type of crossing difficult to predict accurately. Therefore, many students may need to avoid crossing at T–intersections, if possible.

At an offset intersection, this procedure should be used:
• The student determines that the two streets are offset auditorily by listening to the parallel and perpendicular traffic. She then estimates the location of the desired corner and turns slightly toward it to align herself correctly, or she aligns to the sounds of the cars on the opposite side of the street as they idle.
• Once she is aligned, she crosses with the parallel traffic as it first surges forward into the intersection. She adjusts her alignment as she crosses by listening to the moving cars on her parallel street. Depending on the degree of the offset, this can be a difficult crossing to make, even for advanced students. In some instances, students should avoid these intersections, even if it means going out of their way.

Y–intersections should be crossed this way:
• On determining this configuration by listening to the traffic sounds, the student aligns to the perpendicular traffic and crosses one of the three converging streets.
• She does so with each of the streets, as necessary.

PROCEDURES TO CORRECT ERRANT STREET CROSSINGS

The student has the potential to make three basic types of crossings at an intersection. First, she can cross directly to the intended street corner, as was already described (see Figure 8.2a). Second, she can cross while veering away from the intersection or parallel street (see Figure 8.2b). Third, she can cross while veering in toward the intersection. Procedures for correcting the latter two errant crossings, in which the person has strayed from the right course, are described in detail next.

Crossing away from the Intersection

If the student veers away from the parallel street, the instructor remains next to and behind her during the crossing and away from the parallel traffic. The student will inevitably locate her perpendicular street curb and will learn to note three things upon finding it. First, it took her slightly longer to make the crossing than if she had crossed in a straight line. Second, by running her cane along the curb in the street, she notes that the angle of the curb is running not directly across her body, as it should, but slightly diagonal to her; that is, it feels closer to one side of her body than to the other. Third, when she sweeps with her cane to step up onto the side-walk, she notes that she finds grass, not concrete as expected.

To return to her intended sidewalk at the corner, the student does the following:

• She turns toward the direction of the parallel street and corner. She knows which way to turn because the street curb is basically still running across her body and in front of her, so it should still be the edge of the curb of the perpendicular street. Furthermore, she has not turned around or otherwise significantly altered her intended line of travel. The parallel street, therefore, must still be in the same location relative to her that it was before the crossing.

• She uses the three-point-touch cane technique to trail the curb line back to the corner by placing the curb's edge along her side while maintaining the proper direction to approach the corner. The instructor walks along the student's side between her and the parallel cars to act as a buffer, in case cars pass by them.

• She walks along the curb's edge until her cane contacts concrete, which should indicate the street corner.

• With the instructor behind her for safety, the student faces the curb, clears a path with her cane, and steps up onto the street corner.

Crossing toward or into the Intersection

If the student crosses into the parallel street, she is more than likely to cross over to one of five general locations. First, she may just miss the corner and walk slightly into the parallel street, but to the curb on the same corner, as in Figure 8.2c. Second, she may cross the intersection to the diagonally opposite side and to the other side of the parallel street, as in Figure 8.2d. Third, she may cross diagonally to the diagonal corner or to the curb on the opposite of the perpendicular street, as in Figure 8.2e. Fourth, she may cross the parallel street but find the curb on the same side of the perpendicular street, as in Figure 8.2f. And fifth, she may cross the parallel street but find the curb on the opposite side of the parallel street, as in Figure 8.2g.

In each instance, she will know that she has made an errant crossing because the time it took to reach the curb was longer than it should have been had she crossed in a straight line. In addition, she may hear traffic sounds along the wrong side of her or find that walking toward the intended parallel street does not lead her to the intended street corner.

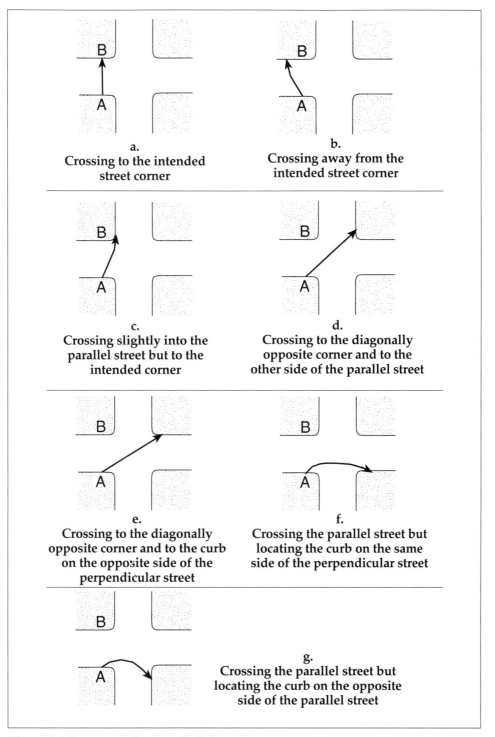

Figure 8.2 Street-crossing possibilities.

As the student begins to veer into the parallel street, the instructor moves toward the parallel cars yet stays closely behind the student. He acts as a buffer and causes the cars to make a wider sweep around the student as they pass by them. This action allows the student to hear the cars on their true side of her and creates a zone of safety for her to respond. Once she realizes something is not right, she should make every attempt to locate a curb as quickly as possible. Generally, if she has walked a longer distance than desired, she can assume she has veered into the parallel street. The sooner she can make this determination, the easier it will be to get back to the curb.

- She turns sharply toward the suspected curb and walks directly to it, carefully noting the sounds of the cars as she walks forward to ensure that she does not walk into their path.
- To determine exactly where she is, the student thinks back to the beginning of the crossing and retraces her route in her mind, noting anything out of the ordinary.
- She listens for sound cues to determine if the traffic is in the right location and, if these cues are available, turns her body to put the sounds in their proper locations.
- She then trails the curb line toward the suspected parallel street until she locates the corner; then she steps up onto it.
- She uses available landmarks and other clues, like the positions of the sounds of the traffic and location of the sun, to determine on which corner of the intersection she is standing, so she may recross the street or streets to get back on her intended route.

INSTRUCTOR'S INTERVENTIONS

The instructor's intervention during a street crossing is perhaps the most difficult aspect of the O&M teaching process. When to intervene, how to approach the student without causing her undue anxiety, how and where to question the student, and how to teach the student the process of decision making under duress are but some of the issues that the instructor must weigh, decide, and act upon instantaneously.

Generally, the instructor intervenes when the student faces a situation she has never experienced before and does not yet have the skills to make a correct conclusion or decision on which to act. Also, the instructor may intervene when there is a "teachable moment," that is, when an unexpected situation arises and the instructor thinks the student is now ready to learn from it.

When to Intervene and What to Discuss

As the situation occurs, in this case as the student veers into the parallel street, the instructor may intervene just after the student has crossed far enough that she should have realized that she has not yet found the curb of the perpendicular street. In a calm and reassuring voice, the instructor stops the student, ensures that the student does not turn her body to talk with him, and asks her if she notices anything unusual about this particular crossing: Has she noticed that she has not yet found the curb? If so, what may be happening to her? Where may she be? Where, then, may the desired corner be to her? And, what does she need to do, therefore, to get back to that curb? He motions any traffic to go around them, if feasible, during this questioning process because the sounds of traffic can help the student determine exactly where she is in relation to the intersection and which way she is facing. The student learns to make rational, timely judgments during moments of high stress, which she will inevitably face when traveling alone in the future.

After the student reaches the curb and steps onto the corner, the instructor congratulates her for successfully reaching her destination, and they discuss the positive aspects of the situation. The culminating question for the student to be asked, and for the student eventually to ask herself, is why she veered in the first place. The student must be able to determine the reason for her veering herself, so she can correct the problem to lessen the likelihood that it will happen again sometime. If the student cannot determine the answer through the questioning process, the instructor guides the questions to elicit the correct response. The student must, however, come to her own realization of the correct answer. It does her no good to be told what she did incorrectly, whether it was swinging the cane too far toward the parallel street during the first step off the curb or initially facing incorrectly, or whatever. The instructor asks such questions as these: When was the last time you knew you were right? What might have caused you to veer? Which one of these possibilities seems most likely to be the correct conclusion? Why couldn't the other choices be right?

Retracing the Crossing

Once the student comes to the correct conclusion, the instructor takes her back to the point of origin of the crossing, and, using the sighted guide technique, they walk along the errant route to the destination corner while discussing what happened. They then return to the corner of origin and walk across the street using the sighted guide technique to the destination corner to feel the difference between the correct and errant crossing. Finally, they return to the original corner, and the student makes the correct crossing independently. The instructor follows this procedure as the student makes each possible errant crossing during the course of this and the ensuing units of instruction.

As the student gains proficiency in recovering from veers, the instructor backs off from this approach and allows the student to make her own recoveries without interventions. Over time, the instructor can "read" the student's mind during this process and second-guess what she will do in a particular situation. The accuracy of his second-guessings and the consistency of the student's responses during errant crossings will determine how safe the student is judged to be and how confident the instructor is with his student under these conditions. As both the student and the instructor gain confidence in the crossings, the instructor backs away from her physically to allow her to experience the crossings truly independently. He may position himself directly or diagonally across the street or even several blocks away.

FAMILIARIZATION TO AN ENTIRE NEIGHBORHOOD

As was mentioned earlier, the instructor selects a neighborhood that provides numerous experiences for the student, ranging from simple to complex situations, and that has areas with little traffic and those with heavier traffic and more complex traffic patterns. The "ideal" neighborhood would include a gridlike pattern of 16 to 24 city blocks, including areas with good sidewalks and those with broken-up and missing sidewalks. The street and traffic patterns would include intersections with one-way, two-way, four-way, offset, and dead-end streets and would have both stop signs and traffic lights. The ideal area would be bounded by a small-to-medium-sized business area for a natural transition into commercial travel. Finally, the area would have alleys, driveways, and walkways and a section that could be used for a transfer-of-skills test.

Before the street-crossing unit, the student may have learned to become familiar with a city block, including the location of landmarks midblock and at corners. She may have walked various routes to and from different landmarks within that block. On learning how to cross streets, the student can now extend the block-familiarization procedures into the entire neighborhood. She first uses the procedure after crossing from the original block to the next street corner. She familiarizes herself to this block in detail as she did with the original block (see Chapter 7). She then walks routes to and from landmarks on this new block and between this block and the original block. She continues in the same way with the next two blocks until she has mastered the blocks that make up the original intersection. By this time, she will have thoroughly learned the familiarization procedure, walked routes while maintaining her orientation, and practiced street crossings.

Rather than continue in this manner throughout the rest of the residential neighborhood, the instructor plans routes that encompass as many of the blocks and intersections as feasible, helping the student move from using tactile landmarks to maintain her orientation to using auditory landmarks and other environmental cues and clues. By the end of the unit, the student traverses the area as she would if she had been walking on her own simply to get from one point to another. She should be so thoroughly familiar with the area that it would be hard for her to become lost or disoriented. The instructor can illustrate this fact to her by developing a drop-off lesson in which the student is left at some unfamiliar origin point in an area that is familiar to her, and she must determine her location to meet the instructor at some predetermined destination. If time allows, the instructor can take the student to an unfamiliar residential area and have her learn the area completely independently over a series of lessons, as a transfer-of-skills test. The student is now ready to travel in commercial areas, where she will modify the cane and orientation skills she has learned to this point in her program and adapt them to the nuances of business travel situations.

CONSIDERATIONS FOR EFFECTIVE TEACHING

Practicing Turns

It may be necessary to practice making good turns, whether the student was born with a visual impairment or acquired it later in life or whether she is a child or an adult. In one example of learning to make appropriate turns, the instructor asks the student to turn toward his voice as he stands off to the student's side. The student learns to feel what it is like to turn exactly 90 degrees to either side. She also learns to turn 180 degrees in the exact opposite direction to perform the second procedure for crossing the parallel street, as described earlier. In another instance, the student places her cane vertically to the ground and up against the side of her body in the direction of the intended turn. She then turns to face her cane at midline, which has remained fixed in its original placement. Similarly, to do a 180-degree turn, she places the cane vertically up against her back and then turns to face it at her midline.

Indoors, the instructor uses a number of teaching aids to help the student learn to make acceptable turns. First, he sets four chairs around the student with the backs closest to the student; each chair is positioned directly in front of, behind, and to either side of the student. The student turns to the instructor's voice and then checks the back of the chair in front of her to determine if it is, indeed, directly in front of her; she makes adjustments accordingly after exploring the chair. Later, the instructor removes the tactile reinforcer to encourage the student to memorize the feeling to create a kinesthetic awareness for the turns. Second, the instructor uses other aids, such as heat lamps (for the sun) or fans (for the wind) to create environmental conditions that can be used indoors or outdoors as cues for proper turning. The instructor's ingenuity in creating other situations or aids will greatly enhance the student's ability to turn appropriately.

Outdoor Numbering Systems

Most residential areas have consistent numbering systems, and the student should learn how to make use of them to locate desired destinations by their addresses. Since addresses run in some sequential order from one block to the next in a given area, the student can make an educated guess as to the address of a particular house on a particular block by knowing an address on another block. Often the even-numbered addresses are on one side of the street and the odd-numbered ones are on the other side. For example, if 105 Elm Street is the third house from the corner of Elm and Spruce, then the third house from the corner of Walnut and Spruce (on Walnut and on the same side of the street as the one on Elm) may also be numbered 105. Similarly, should the numbers run from 100 to 199 on one street, the next set on the same street after the intersection would probably run from 200 to 299.

By pairing a known address with landmarks (tactile or visual), the student learns to locate unfamiliar destinations. It is important that she have consistent shorelining cane skills, especially when searching in unfamiliar territories. Inconsistent shorelining skills may lead her to make erroneous assumptions about a particular landmark search, especially in an unfamiliar area—assumptions that may lead her to miss her destination or to question her judgment about her orientation. Usually, the student's cane skills tend to diminish during these exercises, and it is up to the instructor to anticipate such a situation and to provide timely feedback to ensure that the student uses the cane properly.

Students with low vision need to learn where to look for the numbers of houses. Are they painted on the curb alongside the drive or at the walkway? Over the garage door? Next to the front door? Alongside the front door? On a stair step? On a light pole in the yard? Such students may need to scan with their eyes or use a monocular telescope to locate and read house or building numbers.

9

Advanced Outdoor Orientation and Mobility Skills

In this chapter, procedures are described for helping students use the skills learned in residential areas and apply them to travel in commercial environments, rural areas, and special travel situations. Travel in a variety of situations, from a single block of small shops to complex downtown businesses, suburban malls, and rural areas, is covered. In such situations, students may encounter circumstances that cause them to rely on the public for assistance while maintaining their independence and control. This chapter therefore discusses soliciting assistance from the public and goes on to detail self-familiarization techniques used in various indoor and outdoor areas and travel environments.

The instructor helps the student gain proficiency in commercial travel by developing lessons that provide adequate experiences in finding specific stores and locations within these stores. Instructors should be careful not to follow students too closely, so they can experience the variety of situations that occur when encountering the public. In addition, instructors need to provide students with opportunities for self-familiarization in stores, both inside and out, so it will be possible for them to travel to unfamiliar commercial areas by themselves, without the aid of an O&M instructor. Exposure to rural travel and other special types of travel situations, such as how to negotiate alleys and parking lots, is also important.

SMALL BUSINESS DISTRICTS

It is important for the student to ease into commercial travel by experiencing a small strip of businesses along a city block, usually one bordered by a residential area—preferably the residences explored in the previous series of lessons. The lessons would flow naturally, then, from residential travel to travel in a small business area. The types of shops generally found in such a district include small grocery stores, shoe stores, drugstores, post offices, and barbershops or hair salons.

To begin orientation to stores along a shopping strip, the instructor escorts the student using the sighted guide technique or simply walks by his side while he uses his cane along the strip of small stores. She points out various characteristics of the shops along the building line, including the street furniture found on either shoreline: recessed storefronts, welcome mats, flowerpots, overhanging marquees, various textured surfaces on the building facade, any gradients or slopes, benches or shelters at bus stops, parking meters, and the like. She and the student also note the streets bordering the strip, the compass directions, and any other identifiable landmarks. The instructor points out several stores along the strip and ways to identify them in the future by their specific landmarks or position on the block. For example, one store may be identified simply by noting that it is the first store from a particular street corner, alleyway, or parking lot, whereas another store may be recognized because it is the only one with a mat at its entrance.

The student learns to identify landmarks that he can locate himself or that he can suggest as possible landmarks for others to identify for him. He develops his own style of trailing the shorelines with his cane, using adaptations of the two-point-touch technique without calling attention to his cane as he walks along.

SOLICITING ASSISTANCE FROM THE PUBLIC

The instructor takes care not to tell the student the name of each of the stores because she will eventually ask him to solicit help from passersby to locate some stores. To prepare the student for a variety of experiences in dealing with the public and its perceptions of persons who have visual impairments, the instructor initiates a series of role-playing lessons. She may conduct these lessons in an indoor area to control for the environmental elements that may distract the student from learning the procedures. Some instructors choose to Scotchlite™ the student's cane (see Chapter 5) at this point in the program so it is identifiable to the general public.

The instructor points out to the student that some people are uncomfortable meeting persons with disabilities and may prefer not to involve themselves with individuals who have visual impairments. Therefore, they will attempt to avoid any personal contact by not responding to his requests for assistance. To minimize this frustrating experience, the student learns to select locations along the block that will attract the largest number of passersby while reducing the potential for outright avoidance. For example, by standing with his back nearly up against the corner of a building while facing into the intersection of the two sidewalks (and the two streets), the student will ensure that no one will inadvertently pass behind him and that he will be likely to hear a significant number of pedestrians. He will be able to localize the direction of the passing sound sources more accurately and discriminate the footsteps from other ambient sounds. Furthermore, he will seem either to be waiting for someone or to be seeking assistance.

If a pedestrian approaches the student spontaneously, it is less likely that the pedestrian will try to grab hold of him and push him along the sidewalk if the student is in this position than if he was standing in the center of the sidewalk or at the street corner. If he is grabbed, however, he will perform the Hines break (Chapter 3) to ensure that he has control over the situation. He can also position himself somewhere away from the corner of the building and next to the entrance of a store that receives heavy amounts of pedestrian traffic.

To solicit help himself, the student learns how to greet passersby by scanning with his head to "watch" them as they pass by in order to make eye contact. In an assertive but polite voice, he calls out by saying something like, "Excuse me, please, I need your assistance." He avoids using a gender reference because if he is wrong, he may lose contact with that individual. If the person stops, the student moves toward him or her and continues the conversation by saying, "Could you please tell me how to find Blasch's Shoe Store?" Or, "If I continue in this direction (pointing in a particular direction), will I come to Hill and Hill Groceries?" He avoids asking questions that elicit answers that may be confusing. If the person answers, "Go to the right" or "It's that way," he or she may be pointing in a particular direction, such as to the right, which may be to the student's left side. To avoid confusion, the student reconfirms the direction by pointing and asking the person if that is the direction in which he or she is intending for him to go.

After receiving the necessary information, the student attempts to follow the given directions to locate the store. If he has reservations about this information, it may be wise for him to seek a second opinion from another passerby. If the second person reconfirms the initial information, the student may reasonably deduce that it is accurate. If it differs significantly, it may be best for him to ask the second person to go to the store with him using the sighted guide technique, if feasible. If the person cannot go with him, then it is advisable to get a third opinion or to go into a shop and ask a store clerk for directions.

In some instances, it may be preferable for the student to initiate or accept sighted guide assistance or walk alongside the pedestrian, rather than get into a prolonged discussion on how to find a particular store. As long as the student is assured that he is not taking up too much of the passerby's time or taking the person out of his or her way, then it may be permissible to accept the assistance. As they walk to the destination, he asks the guide what stores they are passing and how to identify the intended store in the future. He thanks his guide at the destination and goes inside the store or tells the guide that he is meeting an acquaintance outside the store in a few minutes.

In the meantime, the instructor stays far enough away from the student to allow the experiences to occur. If she stands too close to him and watches or stares at him intently, she will appear to be with him, and fewer people will approach him. Therefore, she stands far enough away so she can monitor the events without calling attention to herself. She stands across the street and feigns window-shopping while she watches her student through the reflection in the glass. Or, she stands on the same block and window-shops while watching the encounters out of the corner of her eye. In any event, she is within earshot to monitor the conversations and thus is able to provide feedback to the student for improving future meetings with the public.

Finally, in advanced lessons the student learns to telephone ahead and ask store clerks for ways he can identify their stores. He gives them some ideas of what would be useful to use as landmarks. He may ask, for example, if a store is on the corner or near the corner and, if it is near the corner, how many doors from the corner it is. If it is midblock, is there a mat at its entrance or some other tactile landmark near the entrance that he can locate? Is there a bus stop nearby? Is the bus stop before or after the shop, when coming from a particular direction? To remember the information he gathers, he may wish to repeat it into a tape recorder as he hears it to reconfirm its correctness with the clerk and for playback at a later time. The student learns to familiarize himself both within the store and outside the store as well. These skills are discussed in detail later in this chapter.

INTERMEDIATE BUSINESS DISTRICTS

After the student has gained proficiency locating stores along a small strip of shops, he may now be ready to locate and use stores in larger, intermediate commercial areas. Such areas are characterized by a number of blocks of small, retail establishments bordered by primary and secondary streets with various traffic-controlled intersections. Both pedestrian and vehicular traffic are heavier than in the small districts as well. In such areas, the student is able to gain a variety of experiences finding numerous types of stores and store configurations. In addition to the types of stores one would find in small business areas, stores in intermediate business areas usually include convenience stores; supermarkets; restaurants; banks; and various types of retail shops, such as jewelry stores, clothiers, hair salons, and florists.

With these establishments come numerous travel challenges and architectural configurations, such as window-shoppers along building lines; alleys and parking lots (discussed later in this chapter); stores set back from the sidewalk with parking in between; parking meters; bus benches and shelters; islands of trees and shrubbery along the sidewalks; periodic outdoor sidewalk sales with rows of tables, milling shoppers, and racks of clothes; aesthetically pleasing but hazardous objects protruding from the building line, including lampposts, awnings, flower boxes, and telephone booths; and terrain of various textures, from typical sidewalk cement to macadam or pebbled surfaces.

The student uses all the orientation skills he learned to this point, along with the variety of cane skills. He uses the sun; traffic patterns, flow, and controls; the names of the primary and secondary streets within and bordering the area; visual, tactile, auditory, and olfactory cues and clues; and features of the terrain. The student uses the touch-and-slide technique to locate curbs at the corners or to seek mats at entryways or slopes. He uses the three-point-touch, the two-point-touch, or the one down and one up-over technique to locate doors flush against the building line. And he uses the two-point-touch, touch-and-slide, or constant-contact technique along the sidewalk between corners.

Parallel Traffic Alignment

Finally, the student learns to walk parallel to the building line without shorelining and pinballing along the widened sidewalks by keeping the traffic on the parallel street at a constant distance from him. He learns to do so along the curb and building lines, depending upon the direction he is going and the flow of the pedestrian traffic. The instructor uses the sighted guide technique to walk with the student on the side closer to the street; they walk parallel to the traffic sounds, keeping them equidistant (thus, parallel) to them. After walking up and down the street together several times, the student travels the block independently of the instructor, receiving verbal feedback from her until he can do it himself with little or no feedback and without pinballing from side to side.

Development of Meaningful Lessons

The instructor develops lessons that enable the student to refine his skills in dealing with the public to find specific stores and specific locations within stores. The student also learns to request help from store clerks to locate areas within the stores and to price or buy merchandise. Furthermore, the lessons are geared to the student's gender, interests, age, and level of skills. For example, the instructor plans lessons for a young woman and an older man in stores that cater specifically to their tastes and interests in addition to stores that are of general interest to people of all ages and both sexes.

In one typical lesson, the young male student might be asked to locate a specific clothing store along a specific block. He might be given the name of the store and asked to price an item for purchase. He would therefore need to seek out assistance in locating the store, enter the store, obtain help from a clerk, and then exit the store. Succeeding lessons might require him to locate a variety of additional stores, to price and even purchase items, and to use self-familiarization techniques with several storefronts to be able to return to them without having to ask for assistance each time. In the sequence of lessons, each lesson would build upon another in complexity and the requirements for locating numbers of stores, dealing with store configurations (indoors and outdoors), and locating public assistance. The more that lessons are designed to develop a student's ability to seek public assistance, the better prepared the student will be to use this valuable resource. In this way, students become more at ease in various situations and may begin to enjoy interactions with the public in these circumstances.

LARGE BUSINESS AND DOWNTOWN DISTRICTS

These lessons often build upon those developed for small and intermediate business travel areas. The areas discussed here are larger and have a greater number of buildings. The traffic is usually heavier than in smaller business areas and often includes trucks, buses, taxis, and streetcars, as well as passenger cars. In many cities travelers also find subways, loading docks and ramps, and newspaper stands or kiosks. The sounds of the city are louder and more confusing, often punctuated with honking cars and the sounds of construction work, such as jackhammers. The buildings are larger, which often causes wind drafts within blocks, between buildings, and at corners. The types of businesses found in downtown districts include banks, government offices, libraries, post offices, court offices, cultural centers and complexes, parks, and indoor-outdoor malls. Because not all students need to travel in downtown areas, the instructor determines whether to teach this unit on the basis of the student's needs.

In these areas, the student learns to cross streets with a variety of traffic controls, including walk/don't walk signals; traffic islands; police-controlled intersections; and, perhaps, traffic lights with beepers or buzzers to signal when it is safe to cross, which are all briefly discussed next. As the student gains proficiency, the instructor pulls back away from him to allow for natural encounters with the public. During the course of instruction, the instructor may be near the student at the beginning of the unit and several blocks away by the end of it. Culminating lessons include solo or independent lessons (see Chapter 11) in which the student travels alone, locates various destinations, and returns to the agency or school to have the instructor debrief him on the experience.

Walk/Don't Walk Signals

Generally, the student treats walk/don't walk signals as he would any traffic light-controlled intersection, in that he uses the parallel traffic sounds to cross safely and correctly. In some instances, the cycle includes an "all quiet" period in which the traffic is completely stopped on all streets to allow all pedestrians to cross simultaneously. The student uses this period after analyzing the traffic pattern and upon determining exactly when it occurs in the cycle. Some walk/don't walk signals have push buttons to trigger the signal (for further discussion about these buttons, see Chapter 8). The student should never allow pedestrians to tell him when it is safe to cross unless they are willing to escort him using the sighted guide technique. However well-intentioned they may be, pedestrians can only be responsible for themselves and the student can only be responsible for himself when walking separately from one another.

Traffic Islands

Traffic islands are areas in the center of extremely wide streets through which vehicles do not drive. They are generally raised cement areas with curbs, but they can simply be designated areas bordered by painted stripes. If they are elevated areas, the student detects them with his cane as he would in locating the opposite corner, and follows the same procedure to step up onto the elevated area. He may realize that his crossing was completed sooner than expected or may have heard perpendicular traffic in front of him as he stepped up onto the island, so that he would then stand and listen to the traffic patterns. If it is indeed an island, he will eventually note traffic passing in front of him, in which case he completes the crossing during one of the next set of cycles. He, therefore, makes two complete crossings instead of just one.

Police Officer-Controlled Intersections

Although not so common as in the past, there are still areas in which traffic is controlled by a police or traffic officer. The student treats such intersections as if they were controlled by traffic lights. However, on occasion the officer may shout to the student that it is safe to cross. The student is advised never to take anyone's word (including a police officer's) that it is safe to make the crossing. However well-intentioned these individuals are, they may not see oncoming traffic behind them, they may underestimate the time the student needs to make the crossing to dodge approaching vehicles, or they may be shouting to someone else. If the student accepts another person's word, he should be prepared to ask that individual to make the crossing with him using sighted guide assistance.

Beeper or Buzzer-Controlled Intersections

Occasionally, some students may encounter traffic-light-controlled intersections that use beepers or buzzers to alert the pedestrians when it is safe to cross. The student must listen to the traffic pattern to judge which auditory sounds signal which street's cars. The student must not rely solely on the beepers or buzzers in that they may not be working consistently. The safest measure to use in determining the right time to cross is the traffic sounds themselves.

MALLS

Outdoor Pedestrian Malls

Although no cars or other regular vehicular traffic is allowed in outdoor pedestrian malls, occasionally one will encounter special vehicles that are used to make repairs or to transport goods or materials within the mall area. Often the architecture of such malls is aesthetically pleasing, but the design creates particular challenges to persons with physical impairments. The malls can be characterized as having various types of surface textures; blended curbs for wheelchair users; architectural features, such as wide-open sidewalks, gas or electric streetlights on posts, and benches; bus stop shelters along the periphery; alleyways; perimeter parking lots; flower or tree planters; ramps or level changes; and sculpture, kiosks, map and other signage areas, and the like.

The instructor shows the student the overall configuration of the mall by drawing a map on his hand or back or by developing a tactile map of the area. They walk through the perimeter of the mall using the sighted guide technique and begin to locate various stores either by known landmarks or by getting assistance from the public.

SELF-FAMILIARIZATION TO THE OUTSIDE OF A STORE

The student learns to become familiar with the outside of the store, so he can return to it in the future unassisted, using the following procedure:

- He locates the entrance to the store and becomes familiar with its features, as he has done with rooms in indoor settings.
- He then explores the storefront on both sides of the doorway while noting any unique features or characteristics. He estimates how far down the building line to explore by going to the adjacent entrances or by judging the distances. The instructor provides adequate and timely feedback throughout the exercise.
- He then returns to the entranceway and crosses directly to the outside shoreline to begin exploring that area, which he may encounter as he approaches the store in the future.
- He selects a direction to explore and estimates the same distance from the point of origin as he has done from the doorway on the inside shoreline. He notes any objects that may be used as landmarks and then crosses back over to the building line to determine which objects are opposite which ones on their respective shorelines.
- After returning to the entranceway, he recrosses over to the outside shoreline and explores in the opposite direction, crosses back over to the building line, and returns to the entranceway (see Figure 9.1).

The student has thus created an imaginary rectangular "box," with the building line and its opposite shoreline serving as two sides of the box and the respective imaginary internal-external crossover lines as the other two sides of the box. Thus, the explored area has become nothing more than a new "room."

The instructor may wish to introduce this procedure earlier in the outdoor unit and use it continuously throughout the unit as the student moves into different outdoor areas. The student is expected to use the procedure when he is introduced to an area and locates a new store, and he is expected to share the results of his explorations with the instructor at the end of each lesson. By the end of his pro-

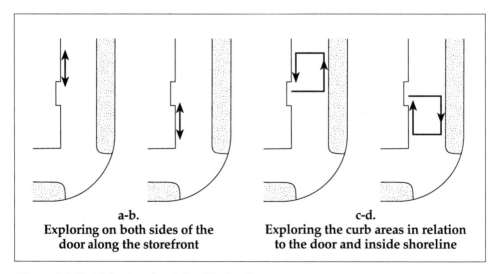

a-b.	c-d.
Exploring on both sides of the door along the storefront	**Exploring the curb areas in relation to the door and inside shoreline**

Figure 9.1 Outside storefront familiarization.

gram, he will have had ample practice in the self-familiarization procedure to have developed confidence in his own travel abilities when negotiating unfamiliar areas.

SELF-FAMILIARIZATION TO THE INSIDE OF A STORE

Self-familiarization to the inside of a store can also be introduced earlier in the outdoor unit. The instructor starts with a small one-room store, usually a specialty shop, and progresses to more complex environments, depending on the particular unit of instruction at that time. A sample progression may be familiarizing from a drugstore, to a shoe store, to a convenience store, to a small restaurant, to a grocery store, and finally to a department store.

Although it is not necessary to describe each familiarization procedure in detail here (since the process is the same as for other indoor environments), it should be noted that as the complexity of the configurations of each indoor environment increases, the familiarization procedures become more complex, similar to room, floor, and building familiarizations. That is, each area is taken one at a time and broken down into its component sections and then "reassembled" into its totality by the end of the process.

The student modifies his cane skills to avoid knocking over items or displays. He can place his free arm behind his back as he walks down crowded aisles to avoid bumping it into people and displays as he might if it was hanging loosely at his side. He can use the constant-contact cane technique to avoid drawing attention to himself, and he can trail carpeted areas to travel alongside display racks in department stores. He keeps track of his cardinal directions as he is led into and through the indoor area, so he will be able to direct himself out of the store after making his purchases.

Indoor Malls

Indoor malls, whether on single or multiple levels, are treated like any other indoor travel area, except on a grander scale. These malls combine the travel challenges of complex and heavily traveled indoor areas with those of outdoor business travel environments. The student will find milling shoppers, noisy environments, interesting architectural configurations, varied stores and storefronts, and a multitude of sensory impressions. Traveling through indoor malls offers many consistencies on which to rely: consistent sound sources, whether from a fountain, an escalator, or a record store; consistent smells and odors emanating from shoe stores, the popcorn vender, the pet shop, or the pizza stand; and a consistent ambient environment in that the "weather" is a constant nonfactor and will not mask sounds or smells. Thus, the student generally knows what he is up against when he enters a particular mall except when special shows, displays, or exhibits may inhibit his ability to use the cues and clues he has relied on during previous visits.

The instructor provides the student with either a tactile map or model of the mall or draws the mall configuration on the student's hand or back. They walk through sections of the mall together and then the student locates various stores and sections semi-independently. He incorporates all he has learned to this point in soliciting assistance to find stores and to locate specific departments and clerks within stores. He uses self-familiarization procedures for stores he will wish to use in the future.

One of the student's greatest challenges may be to negotiate the parking lot to reach the mall itself if he hasn't been driven to the mall and dropped off directly in front of his destination. However, the procedure for traversing all parking lots is the same, and negotiating parking lots will be discussed later in this chapter under Special Travel Considerations.

The instructor provides the student with several different mall experiences so he learns to travel in a variety of mall configurations and to familiarize himself independently to an entire mall. At this stage in the student's program, the instructor's main roles are to expose the student to a variety of travel experiences, observe his behavior, and provide feedback. This is not to minimize the instructor's role in this part of the O&M process, however. Rather, as the O&M program nears completion, the instructor compares the student's skills from the onset of his instruction to the present and evaluates his travel abilities to predict how he will fare as an independent traveler in the not-too-distant future.

TRAVEL IN RURAL AREAS

Often considered the culmination of the O&M program by O&M instructors, rural travel offers unique challenges to the traveler with a visual impairment. Not all students may need to learn to travel in extremely rural areas. However, some environments within or near cities offer experiences similar to those encountered in such areas. In these environments, the student travels vast expanses of open spaces with few distinct boundaries and few auditory and tactile clues or cues to maintain his orientation. He relies upon time-distance estimations and sensory input unique to rural environments. The sun; changes in terrain; distant sounds, such as the tinkling of cowbells and the mooing of cows; the hum of large power-transformer stations; the ringing of church bells; and the roaring of trains and tractor engines all provide information to the student as he navigates through an area. The time of day and the weather conditions (including the direction of the wind) may affect the interpretation of these important tactile, sound, and olfactory clues. Other characteristics of rural areas or similar environments are their unique smells, such as of fertilizer, wet hay, and farm animals; their lack of sidewalks; and the presence of few consistent traffic sounds (except those along a bordering highway).

Because of the unique challenges, the student uses highly developed cane and orientation skills to navigate through rural areas. However, the instructor may occasionally have to introduce rural travel early in the student's program because of time constraints, the student's goals, or the need to conduct lessons in the student's home environment. In those situations, the instructor modifies the recommended sequence of instruction, outlined in earlier chapters, to meet these needs.

The student learns to use modified cane skills to shoreline various features of the terrain, including culverts and other ditches, trails and pathways, pastures, and rocky roads. He uses the touch and-drag technique along culverts and ditches and the constant-contact technique on trails and pathways, through pastures, and along rocky roads. He may learn to use these "modified" techniques as his preferred cane skills if he is learning to travel primarily or solely in his home environment.

The Bundu Basher cane, recently developed in South Africa, offers an alternative cane tip for navigating on uneven terrain (see Resources). The tip is U-shaped, so it does not snag and glides more easily along the surface for ultimate tactile feedback. Marshmallow, mushroom, and teardrop tips also allow for easier gliding than does the traditional cane tip. If the instructor knows in advance that her student will need to learn to travel in rural environments, she would then prescribe one of these alternate cane tips at the time she issues the cane to her student.

Often, there are no discernable clues to use to maintain one's orientation in a particular rural area. In such cases, the student creates his own landmarks. Strategically placed boulders or rock and stone formations cue him to turn down a desired path. A clothesline may connect the farmhouse with the barn, an especially useful device during adverse weather conditions, such as tornadoes, snowstorms, and sandstorms.

SPECIAL TRAVEL SITUATIONS

The following is a discussion of special travel situations that may arise in any of the outdoor units of instruction described in this and the preceding chapters. Because they could be encountered at any time in the residential, business, or rural environment, they are discussed here so that the instructor does not expect them to occur solely in one unit or another. Other special situations are discussed in the next chapter.

Streets without Sidewalks

In most rural areas (and in many suburban areas) travelers must walk in the streets because there are no sidewalks. In these instances, it is preferable for the student to walk facing the oncoming traffic so the drivers can easily see his long cane, which denotes that he is visually impaired. By facing the oncoming traffic, the student is also better able to detect and localize the traffic sounds to make any necessary adjustments in position along the shoreline. If the sounds seem too close, he can step off the street or highway and let the cars pass by. He can also stop walking and pull the cane up close to his body or continue to walk with caution. The student uses the touch-and-drag technique or a modified two-point-touch technique along the textured surfaces of the road and shoreline. The student learns to plan routes so he will be facing the oncoming traffic after each street crossing. If the destination is near a crossing that would not have him facing the oncoming cars, it is acceptable for him to travel on the "wrong" side of the street for short stretches.

As the student approaches an intersecting driveway or road, he notes when the shoreline begins to curve away from him. He then chooses one of two methods to make the crossing. First, he can follow the curve around until it straightens out again. At this point he can square off to the shoreline and make the crossing in a straight line to the other side. Second, he can stop just when he feels the shoreline curve away from him, align to the shoreline, and cross at this point. The former method is a shorter crossing to make, but the student must be careful not to go so far around the curve that he is no longer positioned at the corner. In such a situation, drivers would not necessarily be prepared to brake for a pedestrian and may already be accelerating around the turn. The latter method, on the other hand, is a much longer crossing to make, and the student could find himself in the parallel street. In either case, the student must learn to shoreline effectively to detect the turns, especially if the shoreline is ragged or uneven.

If the student needs to cross a highway without traffic controls, he finds a location that is acceptable, even if it is not at a street corner, and crosses when there are no near traffic sounds. The instructor helps the student discriminate between sounds to be attended to and those that are too distant to be concerned about.

Alleyways

Alleyways are informal paved, dirt, gravel, or mud roads usually found in between streets. They usually run behind houses or businesses. They can be bordered by curbs along the sidewalks, or they can blend in with the sidewalks. They are usually narrower than are typical streets. Upon detecting an alley, the student may not have yet determined that it is, in fact, an alley. Clues that he has come upon an alley may be the shorter-than-expected distance walked from the previous corner, the absence of intersecting sidewalks or other landmarks, the change in the surface texture of the drop-off area, the absence of traffic, and the shorter distance traveled to reach the opposite curb. He treats the suspected (or unsuspected) alley as a street and crosses it using the previously learned street-crossing procedures.

Parking Lots

Parking lots come in all shapes, sizes, and configurations. To learn how to recover his intended line of travel after inadvertently veering into a parking lot as he walks along a sidewalk, the student is escorted into a lot by the instructor and asked to listen for moving cars in the lot and in the bordering street or streets. After the student can discern the difference in the sounds of traffic within and outside the lot, he learns to exit the lot by walking parallel to the traffic sounds along one street until he locates a shoreline to trail back to the sidewalk or by walking directly toward the sounds of the cars in the street and estimating when he has found the sidewalk so he can turn to put those cars along his side. As he detects parked cars with his cane, he learns to explore the angle at which he detects the cars and trails around them using the two-point-touch technique to their opposite sides to square off or align to continue on his intended path. He further uses the upper hand and forearm technique as he trails around a car or truck to detect protruding objects. He uses any combination of these skills and procedures to walk from the sidewalk to an intended destination (building) in the parking lot, or vice versa. The instructor chooses small lots to initiate the procedures and progressively larger lots as the student gains proficiency and as the unit of instruction warrants.

Gas Stations and Convenience Stores

If the student wanders into a gas station or convenience store while walking along the sidewalk, he handles the situation the same way as he handles the general parking-lot procedure. The instructor may wish to escort the student into the station and show him the gas-pump islands, the rubber strips that activate bells when cars run over them, and the buildings. The pump island and the building are used for directional purposes to exit the area. In addition, to maintain his direction as he walks along the sidewalk to avoid walking into the area or off the driveway and into the street, the student uses the touch-and-drag cane technique to shoreline along the seam between the sidewalk and the driveway. If there is constant traffic, the student also maintains his direction by keeping the traffic sounds parallel to him as he walks. He is also careful to listen for cars turning into or exiting gas stations or convenience stores.

Railroad Crossings

If the student is in a rural area or a small town, he may have to learn how to negotiate railroad crossings in a safe and efficient manner. He might realize he is approaching a railroad crossing by the flapping sounds of the car tires as they cross over the tracks, by the rise in elevation as he nears the trestle, by the sounds of the oncoming train, or by the sounds of the warning bells.

As soon as the student hears the warning of an approaching train, he positions himself well back from the tracks and waits for the train to pass the crossing completely. He knows it is safe to cross when he no longer hears the train after it has passed by and when the cars resume their pattern of crossing the tracks. He can also position himself next to the gate, so the gate is between him and the train, and listen for the gate to rise to allow traffic to pass across the trestle.

He detects the tracks with his cane and maintains a straight line of travel directly across the tracks and trestle. He cautiously steps over each track while using the touch-and-drag technique along the trestle edge, which is off to one side. He learns that crossings have at least two tracks and that the usual crossing has at least four tracks for trains going in both directions simultaneously.

CONSIDERATIONS FOR EFFECTIVE TEACHING

Persons with Low Vision

Individuals who have residual vision will build upon the visual skills they have learned in previous lessons and units of instruction. They may locate visual (and in some cases nonvisual) landmarks, identify the streets visually or with low vision aids by reading the street-name signs, and then locate particular addresses and names of stores. To aid in their initial orientation to a business area, many people with low vision develop their own low vision maps or tape-record information about an area for future reference.

Children with Visual Impairments

All children need exposure to business travel, even by going into areas using sighted guides. They need to understand how to shop, how to interact with the public, and how to find and walk through stores. As children grow older, more and more responsibility is placed on them to telephone store clerks to elicit information on how to find stores, to walk to stores or take a bus or taxi to stores, to enter and exit stores, and to purchase items by themselves. Older children with the appropriate skills may receive "clearance" from their mobility instructors to go shopping independently after school hours. Mobility clearance is an excellent motivational tool for mobility lessons (for more information about mobility clearance, see Chapter 11).

Unit Three
ADDITIONAL CONSIDERATIONS FOR THE INSTRUCTOR

The previous section of this book dealt with travel in and through various business and rural areas. In Chapter 10, procedures for negotiating special travel situations are described. These situations include using escalators, elevators, and revolving doors; traveling in adverse weather conditions; using various modes of public transportation; and using electronic travel aids especially designed for travelers with visual impairments. Becoming knowledgeable about numerous types of long canes, including folding or collapsible canes, is also covered in this chapter.

Effective instruction generally involves the use of a variety of teaching approaches with students. Chapter 11 discusses such approaches as O&M survival kits, small- and large-group seminars, tactile maps, auditory maps, and drop-off and solo lessons, as well as the importance of involving others, including the student, in the O&M program.

Chapter 12—the final chapter—addresses certain professional issues: protecting the confidentiality of clients, the O&M code of ethics, and the responsibilities of instructors. Finally, instructors are reminded that they neet to engage in lifelong learning, through continuing education courses offered by professional associations, attendance at conferences, and pursuit of advanced degrees. It is noted that professional O&M instructors have an obligation and responsibility to share their knowledge and expertise in presentations at conferences and workshops and in contributions to the professional literature.

10

Special Situations and Conditions and Mobility Devices

This chapter explores many special situations that travelers with visual impairments confront. Procedures are described for negotiating escalators, elevators, and revolving doors in a safe and efficient manner. Furthermore, general principles and processes covered in previous units of instruction are applied to travel in taxis, city buses, subways, trains, and airplanes. Because it is not possible to travel only in fair weather, techniques for moving through environments under adverse or inclement weather conditions are also outlined. Finally, the many modes of personal transportation that are available in today's marketplace are discussed.

SPECIAL TRAVEL SITUATIONS

Escalators

Two rules are used for negotiating all escalators. First, the metal or wooden plate just in front of the moving steps can be detected with the cane and used for orientation purposes. Second, whatever direction one is facing when stepping onto an escalator will be the same direction when one is stepping off it.

To detect an escalator:

- The student cautiously walks up to the sound of the escalator using the touch-and-slide cane technique while being careful not to trip those in front of her. She first determines whether the escalator steps are moving toward or away from her.
- As her cane tip slides along the metal or wooden plate just in front of the escalator, she listens to the sounds of the escalator. If the sounds of the moving steps are head height, the escalator is either going up and away from her or down and toward her from the next floor above.
- She continues using the touch-and-slide cane technique to locate the moving stair steps and verifies tactually with the cane tip which way the steps are moving in

relationship to her body. If she is still unsure, she sweeps her cane to either side to locate a handrail and lightly grasps it to determine the exact direction in which the escalator is moving. If it is moving toward her, she moves away from it to allow oncoming travelers safe exit. If it is moving away from her, she determines if it is going in the desired direction, up or down. She does so with her cane tip lightly extending over the lip of the metal plate: if it bounces up, the escalator is going down, and vice versa.

- She further notes the cardinal compass direction that is in front of her because it will be the same direction she will be facing once she comes off the escalator on the next floor.

To use ascending escalators:

- The student stands with her toes on the lip of the metal plate, holding the cane in the dominant hand, vertically to the floor, in the pencil grasp of the diagonal cane technique and with the tip between and even with her feet. The student is now ready to step onto the escalator. She allows the cane tip to rest lightly on the moving stairs so it jumps slightly as the edge of each step moves away from her. This position allows her to develop a rhythm so that she will step onto the escalator without stepping onto a moving stair edge and lose her footing.
- After she gets the rhythm of the steps, she places her free hand lightly on the railing and grasps it firmly while stepping forward onto the escalator. She may switch the cane from the pencil grasp to the index finger grasp of the diagonal cane technique (or retain the pencil grasp) with her nondominant foot on the step below her dominant foot and with the cane tip on the step just above her dominant foot. The hand holding the railing is held as far out in front of her as possible to give her advance warning when to step off the escalator.
- As she gets to the top of the escalator, the cane tip will begin to move in relation to her body and the hand holding the railing will feel the railing level off. As the escalator ride ends, the cane tip will hit the plate and her feet will be propelled off the escalator.
- As her feet step onto the plate, she switches to the two-point-touch cane technique and sweeps to clear the area in front of her from the nondominant to the dominant side.
- She quickly steps forward and slightly to the right while using the two-point-touch technique, so she is out of the way of those who are behind her.

To use descending escalators:

- The student locates the escalator with her cane tip; inches forward onto the plate so her toes are at its edge; and checks the rhythm of the moving steps, as she did for ascending escalators.
- She places her dominant hand on the cane in the pencil-grasp position of the diagonal cane technique, grabs the railing with the other hand, and steps forward onto the escalator.
- She switches to the index finger grasp of the diagonal cane technique with the tip resting on the step below her dominant foot. The dominant foot is one step below

the other foot, and the hand holding the railing is held as far as possible in front of her body.

• As the student nears the end of the escalator ride, the cane tip will rise up and the hand holding the railing will appear to level off. She will be propelled off the escalator onto her dominant foot, and at the same time will sweep to clear the area in front of her and exit using the two-point-touch cane technique while walking slightly to the right.

The instructor provides the student with a variety of opportunities to use escalators with various amounts of pedestrian traffic to ensure ease and grace of movement on and off escalators. He also provides the student with different routes on several floors of buildings using escalators, so she learns to maintain her orientation throughout while locating practical objectives.

Elevators

Elevators are usually found near the main entrance to a building or along a back wall of a department store. They may be configured with one door opening to a side or two doors opening out from the center and may be positioned with several banks or rows of other elevators. Usually, summon or call buttons are positioned at waist height and in between elevator doors if there are two or more sets of elevators. Some elevators have bells that ring at each floor, some have automated voices that notify passengers of the floor that is reached, and some have braille or other tactile labels on the button panel, the edge of the door, or the wall just outside the door.

Call buttons can be the kind that are to be pushed or depressed inward or that are heat sensitive and need only to be touched. With heat-sensitive buttons, the student should know that inadvertently touching the recessed button hole can activate the mechanism and that such buttons may not work if she touches them while wearing gloves.

Buttons on the exterior of elevators will indicate either up or down directions: Single buttons indicate that only one direction is possible, as determined by what floor the student is on; if there are two buttons, the top button indicates a call for an elevator to go up, and the bottom button indicates a desire to go down.

Within the elevator, buttons are usually configured in a single column or in double columns, with the lower floors at the bottom of the columns. Even- and odd-numbered floors are separated by columns or alternate between columns. Some buttons, either at the top of the columns or at the bottom, are used to open or close the doors or to trigger an alarm. Furthermore, some elevators have telephones or intercoms to alert the building maintenance department of a failure or fire.

To summon an elevator and locate the correct floor:

• The student presses the desired button and positions herself between elevators on the same wall or facing sideways between elevators on opposite walls. She wishes to position herself so she easily hears and localizes which elevator door is opening. Some elevators have bells with distinct pitches for cars that are going in different directions.

- The student cautiously approaches the open elevator using the two-point-touch cane technique. She shortens her cane length by choking down on the grip to gain better control of the cane, to lessen her chance of tripping exiting passengers. Using her cane skills, she enters the elevator from the right side to go with the flow of traffic and ensures that the elevator is, in fact, there even though the doors have opened.
- After she locates the call panel on either side of the elevator door, she gently runs her fingertips along the buttons to judge the configuration of the numbering system and depresses the button she estimates to indicate the desired floor. If another passenger is in the elevator, she avoids guessing and asks for assistance. If anyone enters during the ride, the student asks for verification of when to exit at the desired floor.

If she is alone in the elevator and no other passenger gets on during the ride, the student must determine the correct floor independently:

- If the button is the kind that depresses and stays depressed, she keeps her finger lightly resting on the button until it pops out, indicating that the elevator has arrived at the desired floor.
- If the button pops out after it is depressed, she keeps her finger on it and depresses it again after the door has opened and then begins to close. If the door opens again, she has reached the desired floor; if it closes and the elevator continues to go, she has probably not yet reached the desired floor.
- If the button is heat sensitive, she keeps her finger close to it and follows the same procedure just described for buttons that pop up.
- If the student is unable to determine satisfactorily the correct configuration of buttons, she estimates where the desired floor button should be and presses a button, exits when that floor has been reached, and seeks assistance to verify the floor number from someone on that floor or attempts to locate a braille or other marker near the elevator.
- As a last-ditch alternative to any of the foregoing procedures, the student presses all the buttons and counts the floors each time the door opens. This procedure is especially inefficient in a large, high-rise building and should be avoided, if possible.

Revolving Doors

Students first learn to negotiate stationary revolving doors before they learn to use revolving doors that are in motion. The following procedure is used:

- The student locates the door either from the side or from directly in front. She prefers to locate it from the right side and to trail the building line to the opening. Because revolving doors generally rotate counterclockwise, it is safer to approach them from the right, since people will exit from their right (or the student's left) side.
- Using the diagonal cane technique, the student locates the door's edge with the cane. She then extends her cane into the opening until it finds one of the four stationary revolving doors. The doors emanate from a center pole or post to form an

X, if viewed from above. Each door has a horizontal crossbar positioned approximately at waist height; the vertical door edge has a rubber strip that flaps against the door wall and outside edges as the door revolves around its circular path.

- The student holds on to the crossbar with the left hand and holds on to the cane with her right hand. The cane is held such that the tip glides along the base of the wall to her right. The student pushes the door counterclockwise until she feels a rush of air or the cane tip detects the opening.
- When the tip finds the opening, the student switches to the two-point-touch technique and exits the revolving door, stepping quickly to her right and out of the way of those who are behind her.

If the revolving door is in motion, the student will hear the rubber edges flapping against the side walls and people moving in and out of it. She localizes the sound and goes to the right of the door to trail cautiously back to the moving door and uses the following procedure:

- At the wall edge, she positions herself so she can touch the edge with her fingertips and feel the rubber edges of the doors as they flap by her. She can use a modified upper forearm and hand position for protection by positioning the hand with the palm facing her and with the fingers along the wall edge.
- As the doors go by her, the student determines the rhythm of the doors to gauge the speed.
- When the rhythm is established and the student wishes to enter, she grabs hold of a door and quickly enters and locates and holds the crossbar. She makes sure her cane is out of the way as she judges the speed of the doors and as she enters the revolving-door area. She must avoid the cane's previously being trapped between the door flap and the side wall or tripping outgoing passengers.
- She uses the same procedure described previously to exit the revolving-door area.

PRIVATE TRANSPORTATION

Whatever the mode of transportation, whether an automobile, van, or truck, students learn to become familiar with both the outside and inside of the vehicle. Instructors teach their students how to walk around a vehicle using the two-point-touch cane technique without damaging the exterior and to use the upper hand and forearm technique when trailing parked or idling trucks to detect protruding side mirrors and other potentially dangerous objects. It is important to learn to identify the exterior of vehicles and where one is in relationship to the vehicles because they can be located in parking lots, in streets, or sticking out into sidewalks. Students must quickly identify their locations to negotiate around and pass the obstructions.

It is important for the student to learn how to enter and exit vehicles safely and gracefully. When entering an automobile, for example, she first checks the seat for objects. She uses the upper hand and forearm technique to locate the top edge of the door frame as a reference and for balance when sitting down. She brings her cane into the car after she sits down and places it in the well between the car seat and the door. She exits the car (from the passenger's side) cane first, swings her feet out and stands up, turns and faces the car, and places the cane in her left hand and up against the car as she shuts the door with her right hand. Whichever side she exits from, she places the cane in the opposite hand from the one that shuts the door.

PUBLIC TRANSPORTATION SYSTEMS

Taxis

Many students rely on taxis as their primary source of public transportation because other modes of transportation, such as buses, are often unreliable or inconsistent. However, taxis have their challenges as well.

In some cities, such as New York, students must hail a cab by standing along the street curb, waving to the oncoming traffic, and waiting for a vacant cab to stop to pick them up. This approach is particularly challenging to travelers who are visually impaired in that it is difficult to distinguish approaching cabs from other vehicles.

In other areas, students learn to telephone taxi dispatchers for pickups. They ask the dispatchers to estimate how long they will have to wait for the cabs, approximate duration and distance of the rides, and the fares. Before they enter the cabs, students remind the drivers of the information they have learned from the dispatchers. Any discrepancies should be corrected before the students actually enter the cabs. The drivers should call their dispatchers for clarification of the best possible routes, approximate charges, and so forth in the students' presence.

Students should periodically question the drivers during the rides to ensure that the agreed-upon routes are being taken: What street are they on? What landmarks are approaching? At their destinations, they should question the drivers about the exact locations at which they are being dropped off and where they should go to reach their destinations. The last steps in the process are to exit the cabs and pay the fares.

City Buses

Depending on the city, riding buses can be a safe and rewarding experience or a frustrating and challenging one, especially during peak hours. It is important for instructors to find stationary city buses (at bus barns, maintenance centers, or the ends of routes) to teach their students the inside and outside bus configurations, to role-play bus rides, and to practice the ridership procedures and techniques. Generally, a little preplanning by instructors ensures that they will have adequate time to teach their students to use buses. Contacting city bus managers and explaining the students' training needs are usually all that instructors need to do to gain the managers' full cooperation. Added incentives to cooperate are offers to do ongoing workshops for bus drivers and other employees on proper etiquette when interacting with riders who have visual impairments.

OUTSIDE BUS FAMILIARIZATION

It is important for a student to become familiar with the outside of buses because if she inadvertently makes contact with one while crossing a street or while trying to locate the door, she will know which way to go to get back on track quickly and safely. The instructor guides the student semi-assisted around the outside of a bus while noting the locations of the doors, the wheel wells, the engine in the back, the side mirrors, and the front windshield. The student learns to trail the bus using the cane and self-protection skills and practices identifying exact locations upon initial contact with the bus.

INSIDE BUS FAMILIARIZATION

Although a student may have little occasion to ride anywhere but near the bus driver, the instructor guides her throughout the bus, so if the student ever has to sit near the back, she will know how to exit the bus from the rear. The instructor shows her the door bar to enter the front door, the side bar as it winds to the fare box, the fare box, the driver's seat, the passenger seats that face the aisle and that face the front, seating areas for disabled and elderly people, the side exit door and doorwell, the signal ropes or strips, and the bars and hand straps along the length of the ceiling. The student learns how to handle her cane as she walks toward the back of the bus by using diagonal cane skills to avoid tripping standing passengers or poking seated passengers.

BUS-UTILIZATION PROCEDURES

With the instructor role-playing the driver in the driver's seat and controlling the door openings and closings, the student stands outside the bus as they use the following procedure:

- The student listens for the opening of the bus door, auditorially localizes its location, and cautiously approaches the bus and door.
- After making contact with the door with the cane, the student asks the driver (the instructor, in this case) if this particular bus is going to the intended destination, using the name or number of the bus route, if known. It is essential for the student to ask these questions before she boards the bus to ensure that she is on the correct bus.
- If it is the correct bus, the student uses the diagonal cane technique with the cane in her left hand, holds the side rail with her right hand, and ascends the steps of the bus.
- The hand holding the handrail glides along to the fare box. The student pays the fare with exact change, determined in advance, and asks the driver to tell her where there is a vacant seat nearby. She also asks the driver to let her know when the bus has reached the desired destination.
- The student sits down and positions the rigid cane vertically to the ground, between her legs and feet and resting against one shoulder, so the cane is out of the way of other passengers.

 If this had been a real situation, the student would have telephoned the bus company to find out the approximate duration of the bus ride in minutes, so she could time or estimate the duration of the ride. After about two-thirds of the riding time, the student reminds the bus driver to tell her when the bus has reached her destination. As a backup, she can also ask a fellow passenger to let her know when the destination has been reached. However, she should not rely solely on fellow passengers, because their information may not be accurate. It is imperative that the student periodically remind the driver to let her off, in case the driver forgets or there is a change of driver in the middle of the route.

After several trips to the same destination on the same bus route, the student learns to pick out her own landmarks, auditorially and tactilely. For example, the bus may go under a particular overpass, make a distinct turn, or go over railroad tracks near the destination.

- When the bus reaches the correct bus stop, the student asks the driver in which direction she must go after she leaves the bus to find her destination and exactly where she should go to catch the returning bus. She then locates the stairs using the two-point-touch technique and exits the bus with the cane in her left hand and holding the side rail with her right hand. She is careful to keep the cane tip low to the steps to avoid poking outgoing or oncoming passengers.
- She steps directly off the bus, walks quickly to the curb, and steps onto the sidewalk.

The instructor and student role-play many different scenarios and practice the different contingencies. In one scenario, the "driver" indicates that the bus is not the intended bus, and the student steps back from the bus as the doors close. In another scenario, the "driver" does not tell the student when the bus reaches the destination, and the bus goes on to the next or subsequent bus stops. In this case, the instructor tells the student that since she must walk back to her destination, she must ask the driver the exact route she should follow before she leaves the bus.

In the first lessons, the instructor may assist the student onto the bus, to an available seat, and off the bus, and may sit next to the student and discuss all that is transpiring on the bus run. In subsequent lessons, the student initiates all the procedures, and the instructor feigns being a passenger and sits farther back in the bus to monitor the proceedings. In final lessons, the instructor may follow the bus in his car and meet the student at a designated destination, or have the student complete an entire bus trip solo (see Chapter 11).

In other lessons, the student learns to call the bus company to get the exact information necessary to ride the bus. If the company has brailled bus schedules, the student learns how to read and use them. In some cities, buses stop at designated bus stops. In other cities, however, every street corner is a potential bus stop, so the student must hail a bus by raising and waving her hand when she hears the bus approaching. It is important for the student to practice facing the oncoming traffic, to learn how to discriminate buses from cars or trucks, and to learn how to approach a bus that does not stop directly in front of her and near the corner. Finally, the student may need to know how to transfer from one bus line or route to another. This procedure may include asking the driver for a transfer ticket on entering the first bus; paying the additional fare, if any; and being directed to another location upon exiting the bus to pick up the next bus.

Further compounding variables are the environmental and weather conditions at the time of the bus run. Adverse weather, to be discussed in detail later, and loud noises, such as jackhammers, will affect the student's ability to hear and localize the sounds of approaching buses or other vehicles.

Although these situations can be discussed at length, the only true way to learn to master them is through practice in real situations. Since bus travel often is the primary mode of transportation for travelers with visual impairments in medium-to-large cities, it is imperative that much of these students' remaining lessons be structured around bus travel to and from various sites.

Trains

Unlike buses, trains do not have doors that open and close, but they do have steps and side rails. Each car is a self-contained seating unit, but with no one person who is permanently assigned to that car and designated to provide information. Passengers enter and take their seats. At some point a conductor passes through the cars and collects prepaid tickets or fares from passengers who do not have tickets.

The instructor familiarizes the student with the train station or depot, both inside and out, and the procedure for entering and leaving a train. He shows the student how to detect the platform with her cane, how to walk parallel to the platform, and where to wait for the approaching train. Some train platforms have tactile guide strips that warn pedestrians of the platform's edge and pit and that can be detected by a cane. The student learns how to step up into the train, to find a seat, and to leave the train. Unlike buses, trains only stop at designated stops along a route, so the student can count the number of stops to determine her destination. Also, the conductor usually passes through the cars to announce the oncoming train stops.

Rapid-Rail and Rapid Light-Rail Systems

SUBWAYS

Subways are nothing more than underground trains, although there are different procedures to follow. The student pays for a subway ride with the exact fare or with a token either at a toll booth or as she goes through a turnstile.

One type of turnstile is a configuration of individual rotating, horizontal bars that allow one person at a time to go through, such that a bar rotates into position after one person pushes through and before the next person goes through. This type looks like a revolving door, only with a series of bars positioned horizontally from floor to ceiling. Persons push the "door" and go through one at a time; the door rotates only in one direction. It is important for the instructor to follow the student through a turnstile, rather than precede her, especially if the student changes her mind and decides not to go through. There is nothing more disconcerting than seeing one's student go off in another direction and not being able to follow!

The student learns to walk along the platform and to enter a subway car, which is at the same level as the platform and thus has no stairs to climb. However, there may be a more-than-slight space between the platform and car, so the student learns to use caution and proper cane skills to avoid accidents or injuries. In some subway stations, trains pass along both sides of a platform, so the student learns the direction in which trains are going on each side of the platform and to take precautions when walking along either side of the platform.

Many subway cars are packed with passengers, especially during peak hours, so students learn to hold on to the vertical bars or hand loops and stand during the ride. They must negotiate tight spaces and brace themselves during surges of stopping and starting at each station. Since cars stop at each station, students can count the number of stations to their destinations. Often, the conductor will announce the approaching station on the intercom, although it is sometimes difficult to hear or understand the announcements.

Finally, the student learns to leave the car and exit the station. Because each station in a system and each city's subway system is different, every possibility cannot be described here. However, the instructor shows his student any consistencies among the stations and ways to determine how to exit safely to the street level. For a more detailed discussion of subway travel, see Uslan, Peck, Wiener, and Stern (1990).

ELEVATED TRAINS

Elevated trains, or Els, are negotiated similarly to trains or subways. Often the stations or stops are located by climbing steps to an elevated platform. Students handle the entering, fare paying, and exiting according to the procedures for a particular city.

RAPID TRANSIT AND TROLLEYS

Electrified light-rail systems like rapid transits and trolleys are rail driven with electricity received from overhead power lines. Each city has its own system and procedures to learn and follow. Generally, the systems are intercity and have a limited area of operation. Often, the electric systems tie in with buses, subways, or trains to provide a wider range of coverage.

Air Travel

Airports present a significant challenge to travelers with visual impairments. Finding the airline baggage and check-in counter, negotiating the airport to locate the gate, handling carry-ons, and locating one's seat can be accomplished somewhat independently. However, airlines must follow federal and internal regulations that may restrict a student's ability to handle these challenges alone, even if she wishes to do so.

The instructor teaches the student how to seek assistance at strategic areas of the airport and how to travel through the airport. At the baggage check-in counter, for instance, the student can find sighted guide assistance to travel to and through the metal detectors. If the student alerts the airline of her arrival time at the airport, unnecessary delays in obtaining assistance can be avoided. Also, by allowing additional time for delays in obtaining assistance during heavy traffic periods, the student can avoid a high-stress situation and enjoy a relatively trouble-free experience.

The student who wishes to travel independently will need to learn to travel throughout the airport or, at least, to travel specific routes to various destinations, including rest rooms, restaurants, and waiting rooms. She learns that she will not be allowed to keep her rigid cane at her seat on the plane and thus should be prepared to have a folding cane at her disposal during the flight. Although most airlines today will offer assistance at boarding gates, the student may wish to board the plane on her own. In such instances, she learns that she may need to climb steps to enter the plane or to negotiate stairs to reach a jetway in some airports, that the jetway may lead directly from the boarding gate to the airplane in others, and that she will need to step over the lip of the airplane door from the jetway to enter the plane itself. Once in the plane, flight attendants will escort her to her seat.

ADVERSE WEATHER AND NIGHT TRAVEL

It is difficult to learn skills or to travel safely through areas if students are cold, wet, or hot. Proper clothing minimizes these conditions and enables students to concentrate on their O&M skills. Therefore, appropriate clothing is as essential as are proper canes or other mobility devices and will be discussed in relation to specific conditions. Because it is important for students to learn to travel in all weather conditions, instructors should encourage their students to meet them for lessons at times when the weather conditions are not ideal.

Traveling in Cold-Weather Conditions

Cold-weather conditions include subfreezing temperature, snow, ice, sleet, and wind. Students learn to wear layered clothing, including long underwear; two or more pairs of socks; heavy nonslip shoes, boots, or galoshes; fur or other insulated gloves (the thinner, the better for the best tactile receptivity); shirts; sweaters; and head, face, and ear wear. It is important to be protected from the elements without impairing one's ability to feel the cane and its sensory feedback or to hear ambient sounds, especially traffic noises.

Traveling in snow presents unique challenges. Snow can be soft and powdery, compacted and hard, or slushy, depending upon the temperature and travel location. Students learn to walk on sidewalks, for example, that have compacted snow from many pedestrians trampling over them or soft, powdery snow from the lack of pedestrian foot travel. As they approach the corners, they may find slushy street corners and streets. Thus, students learn to maintain their orientation by understanding the consistency of the snow. Curbs blend in with the streets as snow builds up, and snowbanks are created by snowplows pushing snow onto the corners. Traveling along sidewalks can be fairly easy in the snow because the snowbanks force the students to stay on course. Students use the constant-contact cane technique along sidewalks and learn to step or climb over the snowbanks and into the streets before aligning for the crossing. Students further rely on estimating the distance from one corner to the next because it is difficult to detect curbs under these conditions. Finally, the sounds of cars are muffled by the snow and are often detected only as cars come immediately beside students.

Traveling on ice or in sleet is equally challenging. When they detect icy patches of ground, students learn to widen their bases of support and walk with a slow, shuffling gait while attempting not to raise their feet off the ground, so they maintain as much contact with the ground as possible. At most shoe stores or shoe-repair shops, students can purchase temporary ice cleats to strap onto their shoes or boots for better gripping power. They use the constant-contact cane technique along the icy patches for better feedback.

Traveling with a cold, heavy wind can challenge any pedestrian. It is especially difficult for students to maintain their balance and orientation to the sounds around them. Sounds can be masked or muffled, or the direction and location of their sources can be misinterpreted. Therefore, students learn to rely primarily on tactile cues and clues. To minimize facial freezing and burns, students can wear knit ski masks, as long as they uncover their ears before and during street crossings.

Instructors tailor lessons to fit the weather conditions and students' levels of fitness. Obviously, very young or elderly students will need to take frequent breaks from the cold. Similarly, students with diabetes and, consequently, poor arterial circulation, should not stay outside in extremely cold weather for extended periods. Thus, instructors must gauge the fine line between when a situation may provide an excellent learning experience and when the weather will adversely affect learning.

Traveling in Hot-Weather Conditions

Hot weather places students at risk of heat stroke, sunburn, and other maladies associated with summer travel. Therefore, students should consider wearing light-colored clothing that covers all their exposed body surfaces or should apply sunscreen to exposed parts of their bodies at least 30 minutes before their lessons or outings. Furthermore, students, especially those with diabetes, must avoid wearing sandals on lessons or when traveling independently to avoid stubbing or breaking their toes.

Lessons incorporate periodic breaks to seek shelter from the sun, and students learn to plan routes on shady sides of the streets, whenever possible. Students learn to carry salt tablets and liquids with them to avoid heat dehydration or prostration. Finally, just as tennis players wipe off their rackets after every point when it is hot and sunny, students keep their cane grips and hands as dry as possible when they travel by periodically wiping them with a cloth or towel.

Traveling in Rain

Rainy conditions can be especially challenging to students. Proper rain gear should be worn to keep as dry as possible, especially if it is also cold. If umbrellas are used, students learn how to hold them out of the way or high above their heads when listening to traffic to avoid confusion in auditory localization of the traffic sounds. While walking or standing still, students learn to position the umbrellas between them and the direction of the rain, whether it is directly from above or off to their side. Students must wear water-repellent outerwear, shoes, or rubbers and should carry extra shoes and socks to change into on reaching their destinations.

Often, car sounds are easier to track in the rain because tires splash back on wet pavement and create a "line" of sounds. While some sounds become muffled in the rain, others, like the splashing of tires, can be heard at greater distances for a longer time. However, crossing streets in the rain can be difficult because students must negotiate puddles, water pouring into gutters, cars splashing water on them, and their cane hands becoming soaked, thus decreasing sensitivity. Finally, students should find other ways to travel than by walking if there is a threat of lightning. Because umbrellas and aluminum canes can attract lightning, students should seek shelter from storms as quickly as possible.

Traveling at Night

For students who are totally blind or who have low vision, lessons on night travel should be structured at night. Because sounds are heavier and lighting conditions are different at night than during the day and pedestrians' interactions and drivers' reactions differ significantly at night, blindfold or low vision simulation experiences during daytime cannot adequately simulate nighttime conditions. Therefore, instructors should be compensated for night lessons either by compensatory time or overtime pay. Whenever students cannot receive night travel instruction, instructors note this fact in their reports, because they cannot be sure how well students will adapt to nighttime conditions and situations without such instruction.

OTHER MOBILITY DEVICES

Collapsible or Folding Canes

Many types of collapsible canes are on the market today. Many come with four or five aluminum sections with one or two elastic cords connecting the sections to the tip at one end and the grip at the other. Grips are metal or rubber, and tips are either metal or nylon. Many folding canes have elastic cords on the grip end that are used to bind the canes when folded. Some canes are manufactured with the natural aluminum shaft sections exposed, while others have the standard white and red coatings already applied or baked into them.

Generally, many of the folding canes are well made, and thus students should choose the ones they prefer. Some people prefer canes that fold up as small as possible and, therefore, pick ones that have five small sections, rather than those with four large sections. Some persons prefer canes that break apart easily at the joints, so they choose canes with Teflon-like coatings at the joints and, perhaps, single elastic cords. Others prefer sturdy and rigid-type canes and will choose canes with double elastic cords or metal cables.

Although some students prefer to use collapsible canes as their primary mobility device because such canes are easily stored, they should be aware that each joint in the cane lessens the cane's receptivity and, hence, the user's sensitivity; that is, what one gains with convenience, one loses in usage. However, students should consider carrying a collapsible cane with them for emergency situations when the primary cane is broken and a backup cane is needed. Students learn to keep collapsible canes in an extended, full-length position when storing them to avoid causing undo stress on the cords. They also learn not to place their wrists through the cord loops when using the canes to avoid serious injury if the cane gets stuck in a moving vehicle or they trip and fall. (For a list of cane manufacturers, see Resources.)

Dog Guides

Dog guides escort their owners around obstacles, barriers, and hazards. It is a common misconception, however, that they know where they are going. The dog guide user must direct the dog along the route to the intended destination every step of the way. Only after walking a particular route exactly the same way over extended periods will dog guides seem to lead their owners to a destination without verbal commands.

Dog guides are viable options for those who have extensive travel needs and who do not wish to know everything there is to know about their travel environments, as is the case with long-cane users. Dog guides are preferred mobility aids for a small population of travelers with visual impairments. Students who can walk at a fast pace for extensive periods may be excellent candidates for dog guides because dogs travel at speeds of up to five miles per hour. Since the two must work well as a team, they must practice together for many months so they begin to trust each other's judgments. That is, students must learn to trust that their dogs are, indeed, taking them around obstructions when, for example, they are guided off and then back onto sidewalks. Similarly, dog guides must trust their owners' judgments that they are, indeed, crossing a street at the proper time when given a command to cross. Dog guides can, however, refuse to obey incorrect commands; they are taught to exercise "intelligent disobedience" under certain conditions, such as when cars run red lights.

Instructors must counsel their students on the appropriateness of their interests in using dog guides while not discounting the viability of their decisions. Ultimately, adults have the right to make their own decisions about which mobility aids they will use. Dog guide users should have a good knowledge and understanding of environmental and spatial relationships to make the best use of dog guides, since students with poor orientation skills often prove to be limited travelers, even when using dog guides. Furthermore, students who have severe mobility restrictions, such as wheelchair users, many elderly people, or those who have had strokes or have other physical impairments, should look for other travel options. Once they have decided to use dog guides, students must be encouraged to continue with their O&M training programs. They must build on their orientation skills and develop other mobility options in case their dog guides become sick, disabled, or unusable for a time.

Because they are not professionally trained to teach or correct what appears to be the incorrect usage of dog guides, instructors limit their teaching to orientation skills. If an instructor suspects that a student is mishandling a situation or physically abusing her dog, he should discuss the problem with the student to rectify it as quickly as possible. Persistent problems should be referred to the appropriate dog guide training school.

Electronic Travel Aids

Electronic travel aids (ETAs) are mobility devices that were developed to extend the range of sensory awareness of the traveler with a visual impairment beyond the fingertip, cane, or dog guide. They are generally head-borne or hand-held devices that emit ultrasounds or laser beams to probe the environment and, should objects be detected, alert the users through auditory or tactile sensations. Users of ETAs learn to interpret these signals to determine whether they wish to make contact with or avoid the objects in their paths.

Since the 1960s, many ETAs have been introduced into the market, but only a few have been widely accepted by mobility specialists and consumers with visual impairments. Some ETAs that have gained worldwide acceptance are the Mowat Sensor, the Pathsounder, the laser cane, and the Sonicguide.

The Mowat Sensor is a lightweight, hand-held device that emits ultrasounds and signals the user through vibrations in the unit. Users learn to point the device in the direction of suspected objects. They use it as a complementary travel aid with either a long cane or a dog guide.

The Pathsounder is a chest-borne, complementary ETA that emits ultrasounds into the environment. When the device detects obstacles, the sounds are reflected back into the unit and translated into either tactile vibrations of the unit or neck strap or into auditory sounds. The device is generally used with a long cane or a dog guide or, occasionally, modified to be head-borne and used when sitting in a wheelchair.

The laser cane is a modified long cane that emits three pencil-thin laser beams aimed to extend three feet out to the user's forehead height, 12 to 15 feet out to the user's waist height, and to the ground three feet beyond the cane tip. The beams are reflected off objects and back into the cane. They are translated into tactile and auditory signals, and users learn to interpret each signal in relation to the respective beam.

The Sonicguide is a pair of spectacles with ear flutes that emits ultrasounds into the environment. The device is used as a complementary travel aid with either a long cane or a dog guide. When objects are detected, the signals are reflected back into the spectacles and translated into audible sounds through the ear flutes. Users learn to interpret the distances of detected objects by changes in the pitch of the sounds. They also learn to determine exactly where objects are in their fields of view, or azimuth, by interpreting the binaural or stereophonic effects of the sounds. And, finally, they determine the approximate composition of the objects by the tone of the sounds. Therefore, the Sonicguide is a true environmental sensor for persons with visual impairments. It, as well as all the other devices, requires rechargeable batteries.

In the past, mobility specialists who were trained in using ETAs have studied the ability of these devices to enhance the learning of mobility skills, spatial relationships, and the overall growth and development of infants and toddlers who have visual impairments. Even though their successes in these areas have been well documented in the literature, general acceptance of ETAs has been hampered by their high cost, limited availability, and the cost of training programs. Although manufacturers have recognized the importance of training professionals to use the devices before consumers can make successful use of them, few O&M specialists have been trained to teach the use of ETAs. As a consequence, few travelers with visual impairments have had access to or interest in using them. (For a list of manufacturers of ETAs, see Resources. The requirements for instructor training for ETAs and the availability of current training workshops can be obtained by contacting specific manufacturers or AER, whose address and telephone number are also listed in Resources.)

11

Creative Approaches

Often, the teaching of O&M skills does not simply entail the one-to-one teaching of skills, as described thus far. O&M instructors look for a variety of ways to help their students attain their mobility goals. This chapter explores some of the ways that effective instructors create special learning situations that enhance their students' O&M programs.

As has been emphasized throughout this book, motor and cognitive skills must be taught in a multitude of ways and in a variety of environments for students to believe that they truly understand how to travel safely, independently, and efficiently in all situations. Some approaches that enhance the regular O&M curriculum include drop-off lessons, in which instructors take students to known environmental areas without telling them their precise locations and students learn to determine their locales to get themselves to prearranged destinations. When used judiciously, drop-off lessons prove to students that they can regain their orientation under stressful conditions. Solo lessons, on the other hand, allow students to see how well they trust their travel skills and how well instructors trust their teaching abilities. Students travel to and from destinations without monitoring by instructors and report back to their instructors on how well their experiences went. If successfully implemented, these approaches can boost students' confidence in their travel abilities.

Instructors must find ways to incorporate the skills they teach at times other than during normal lessons. Off-lesson, or homework, assignments place the responsibility of learning and practice directly on the students. These assignments range from independently practicing skills to listening to audio self-instruction tapes. Some instructors have developed computer modules for learning simple to complex spatial and other orientation skills. Others have encouraged their students to develop mobility "survival" kits that remind students how to handle certain complex situations.

The importance of developing cognitive maps of areas has already been mentioned in this text. One way that students learn to develop cognitive maps is by first learning the use of tactile and auditory maps. One type of tactile map is a hand- or computer-developed raised-line representation of a travel environment; using their fingers, students trace along the raised-line images of city blocks, state and federal highways, county boundaries, rivers and streams, and the like. Another type of tactile map is hand drawn on the student's hand or back to depict an immediate travel environment. Such maps are simple and useful learning tools that many O&M instructors incorporate into most lessons. Auditory maps, on the other hand, enable students to listen to taped explanations of detailed descriptions of travel areas. When used together, tactile and auditory maps are excellent tools for learning about and traveling through simple and complex environments. As students gain proficiency in traveling through these environments, they develop a cognitive understanding of the travel areas by visualizing them in their minds and may, therefore, no longer need the maps.

This chapter also explores the multitude of ways to involve students' families, friends, peers, and others who work with them in the mobility-learning process. Observations of lessons by family members and other teachers and friends, small- and large-group seminars, and concept and life-skills classes are a few of the approaches used. By involving all who are important to the students in the mobility program, instructors ensure that skills are encouraged, correctly reinforced, and monitored at all times.

SCHEDULING STUDENTS FOR MOBILITY INSTRUCTION

Finding time in the student's schedule for mobility instruction can be a challenge for the instructor, especially with older students in public schools and schools for the blind. Early-grade and preschool students can be easily scheduled for instruction because they can be taken out of some activities without significantly affecting other skills. As education becomes more formalized, constraints are placed on students' curricula that restrict the freedom to "add on" other nonacademic needs, such as mobility instruction. Although it may be necessary to take a student out of a study hall, gym class, health class, or even an academic class, such situations are less than ideal and deprive students of a well-rounded academic experience.

The author has found that by developing a competency-based mobility curriculum that permeates students' entire academic lives from preschool through 12th grade, it is easier to schedule older students for mobility instruction. In these instances, students are assigned a total number of units of instruction, including 16, 18, or 24 units of mobility instruction, that they must complete before they can graduate from school. Units or credits can be completed quickly if skill levels and age levels are appropriate. For example, credit units may be broken down into the following components: basic skills, cane skills, indoor skills, introductory outdoor skills, intermediate outdoor skills, and advanced outdoor skills. Each unit may be further broken down into subunits, as detailed in this text. As students progress, they receive pass-no pass credit or even grades, if they so desire. In this manner, students would not be taken out of any other classes to receive instruction, since they would be assigned a class specifically for mobility instruction for that semester or year. Students could receive several semesters or years of instruction or not receive further instruction for one or several years and then be picked up for instruction again, if necessary. Obviously, the instructor must "sell" the school superintendent and school board on this approach, which is not an easy task.

STUDENT-CENTERED EXPERIENCES

As was mentioned earlier, drop-off and solo lessons are ways to develop students' self-confidence while they are still under the tutelage of their instructors. In the drop-off lesson, the student is unaware of his point of origin but knows the destination point. The trick is to figure out where he is, or to reorient himself, and then to travel to his destination. The purpose of the lesson is to show the student that although he may become disoriented along a route, he is still capable of reorienting himself without becoming afraid or frustrated or losing control of the situation.

Drop-off Lessons

Instructors generally use drop-off lessons at varying times within the O&M program, usually at the end of the indoor, residential, commercial, and rural units of instruction. To create a real-life feeling of disorientation, the instructor finds creative ways to bring the student to the drop-off site without raising his suspicions, such as by maintaining a distracting discussion and using a heretofore untraveled route to the travel site. At the site, the instructor discusses the purpose of the lesson and how the student can reorient himself. If the destination is many blocks from the drop-off site, the instructor waits for the student to commit himself to a direction after he leaves the car before following behind him or driving directly to the destination.

The student learns to use the available information in his immediate environment for reorientation. Often, by simply walking to a street corner, the student will gain the necessary cues and clues to piece together his exact location. Changes in terrain, traffic patterns, the sun, or specific tactile landmarks may redirect the student to the correct path to his destination. As he builds success in these lessons, the student should gain the self-confidence necessary to overcome the fears associated with being temporarily lost. The instructor's confidence in her feelings about the student's level of skills also increases. Thus, drop-off lessons can be challenging, fun, and confidence building for all concerned.

Solo Lessons

Solo lessons are culminating experiences in the O&M program. However, some instructors use them at the end of various units of instruction to show their students that they can travel independently as they learn their skills for safe and efficient travel. In a solo lesson, the instructor takes the student's perspective into account and asks the student to travel to a particular destination in a known or unknown environment and waits for the student to return to the point of origin. Obviously, the instructor must have a good deal of confidence in the student's travel abilities to trust that he can handle whatever experiences may arise without any intervention.

A common mistake is for the instructor to tell the student that he is going by himself on the route, when she intends to follow him—to make sure nothing dangerous happens to him or just to see what happens along the way. Unfortunately, if something goes awry, the instructor must decide whether to intervene. If she does, she risks losing the trust she has established and betrays her lack of confidence in her student. Thus, it is strongly advised either to make the lessons truly "solo," or to tell the student in advance that the lesson is not really a "solo" lesson in that the instructor will be observing from afar. However, in such a case, the instructor should not delude herself into thinking the student is traveling independently when he is actually traveling under her supervision. Therefore, solo lessons are designed to improve the confidence of both the student and the instructor in the student's travel skills. How else will the instructor verify that her student is, indeed, a safe and independent traveler under some or all situations?

Mobility Clearance

To conduct drop-off and solo lessons or even instructor-led lessons, for that matter, it may be necessary for the instructor to receive permission to teach the student off the school or agency grounds. In some instances, especially at public schools, it may be difficult to do so. Many public school administrators are not familiar with mobility instruction and the fact that learning should occur in natural settings away from the school grounds. They may not see the need for it, especially when the student is functioning well on campus and hence does not seem to need mobility instruction.

In such cases, the instructor may have to work closely with the school superintendent, principal, other teachers, and parents so that all involved may better understand the importance of mobility instruction and the need to go off campus at times. It has been the author's experience that time spent developing these relationships and rapport before the start of the school year is time well spent. Individual and group conferences with the parents, superintendent, and principal and in-services for teachers are integral aspects of mobility instruction—even for one student. In some states, outreach vision programs have developed statewide conferences and workshops that are designed to acquaint teachers and school administrators with the educational needs of their students with visual impairments, including their mobility needs.

Once clearance has been obtained, instruction may have to be initiated and further clearances approved in other public and private settings. Such areas as churches, city halls, private factories, malls, hospitals, and public libraries are just a few of the indoor facilities used by itinerant O&M instructors.

Mobility Passes

One difficult type of clearance for both the O&M instructor and the school or agency administrator is clearance for the student to leave the institution's grounds during off-class hours for personal reasons. But once students have demonstrated consistently safe mobility skills, it is imperative for them to use their skills on their own time. Many instructors issue mobility passes that clear students for such independent travel. Obviously, liability factors must be taken into account by all concerned, but, ultimately, this practice is part of the overall mobility experience. It is far better for students to experience problems in this type of atmosphere, where they still have access to their O&M instructors and can work out the "kinks" in their travel skills, than to experience problems later when they do not have access to O&M instructors.

The O&M Survival Kit

Since O&M instructors cannot be with their students after their programs have concluded, it is necessary for the students to learn to monitor their own skills and solve their own problems. But self-monitoring is challenging without the use of vision. Students have difficulty determining, for example, the reasons why they keep bumping into shorelines or tripping off curbs. Were they using the proper cane skills? Were their hands centered when using the two-point-touch technique? Was the arc height too high to detect the curbs? Why was their alignment off when they crossed a street? To answer these and other questions without the aid of others, students can develop and use mobility survival kits.

These kits are either audiotapes or brailled notebooks that describe in detail the myriad situations that may occur when traveling, the consequences of handling the situations in certain ways, and the options for correcting those situations. Instructors may encourage students to develop these kits from the beginning of their O&M programs. As the students learn skills, they can describe and catalog them in the survival kits, which the instructor reviews periodically for accuracy.

One example of such a notation may be this:

> Whenever I find myself bumping into a grassline each time I swing the cane over to one side, I may be swinging the cane too wide to that side, or my hand may not be centered, or the sidewalk may be curving around to the opposite side of me. Let me try to narrow my arc width and, if that does not work, I will try to center my hand. If neither option works, I will listen to the traffic and see if it sounds like it is curving around me; if I am still unsure, I will realign to the shoreline and then walk forward and slightly away from it.

This notation would be catalogued under "sidewalk travel." It could be further abbreviated by noting: "Keep hitting shorelines—arc too wide? Hand centered? Sidewalk curving?"

Another example may be as follows:

> I keep veering away from the parallel street when I make a crossing. Is it always to the same side, or does it matter? Maybe my hand isn't centered when I step into the street. Or maybe I am not aligned correctly; next time I will pay more attention

to the alignment of my head and feet and adjust them slightly. If that doesn't work, I'll try turning slightly toward the parallel street after I think I'm aligned properly.

An abbreviated notation could be: "Veer away from parallel street—check consistency of direction, hand position, body alignment, and so forth."

When students compile detailed descriptions of problem-solving situations, along with descriptions of techniques and skills, they will have developed a comprehensive mobility notebook. The process of developing the notebooks or kits reinforces the skills as they learn them. By closely and constantly monitoring the kits, instructors ensure that the skills are not misunderstood. Finally, the mobility survival kit becomes an integral tool for learning the skills. It will be useful to students long after they have completed their O&M programs.

Tactile, Auditory, and Hand-drawn Maps

Tactile maps are concrete representations of spatial relationships (raised-line drawings that can be felt with one's fingers) that are beyond the reach of travelers with visual impairments. Usually, they depict the relationship of objects in a room or building, configurations of streets and city blocks, or other complex travel situations (shopping malls, subway systems, and so on). Often, they are made for particular travel routes and may be called "strip maps." In any event, tactile maps are usually easy to make, simple in design, and transportable.

A tactile map can be made at home with few tools. Pipe cleaners or strips of wood can be glued onto a piece of braille paper to represent a sidewalk, a building, or the shape of a route, for example. The map can then be placed on a thermoform machine and used as a master to be copied onto a piece of thermoform paper. The student can then use the thermoformed map without fear of damaging the original.

Another method of mapmaking is using the Tactile Graphics Kit made the by the American Printing House for the Blind (see Resources). The kit contains various tools used to indicate such differences as those between a county and a state border or a river and a county line or to show such elements as the intersection between two roads. The mapmaker carves the lines onto a foil sheet to create a master, which is then placed onto a thermoform machine to make a copy. For a complete description of the mapmaking process, tools, and the like, see Edman (1992).

Auditory maps are more detailed explanations of travel environments. For example, whereas a tactile map may depict the buildings on a college campus and their relationships to one another, an auditory map may go into greater detail about a particular building or set of buildings. Whereas the tactile map may show where a building is located, the auditory map may explain the actual shape of the building, what is located on particular floors, and the exact interior layout. Likewise, an auditory map may provide greater detail of the travel route—the location of landmarks or travel hazards and slopes to note while traveling. By using both tactile and auditory maps, students become well equipped to handle most travel environments with little fear of becoming disoriented. Once an area becomes familiar, students need not carry or use the maps again.

Hand-drawn maps are those made by someone else using his or her finger to draw an area to be traveled on the student's hand or back. Frequently, the drawing is of only the particular route to be walked, but at other times it is a more sophisticated representation of a travel area. It is important to draw the map simply and in the plane in which the student visualizes it. For instance, some people visualize an intersection of streets as if they were looking at a map on a table top, that is, by looking out from the body in a horizontal plane. Such representations would be better visualized by drawing the map in the palm of the hand, which is held out in front, palm up and parallel to the ground. Others may visualize best as if they were looking at a map on a wall, that is, in a vertical plane. Thus, they may better visualize a hand-drawn map on their back, using the same plane of view. Obviously, hand-drawn maps must be made simply and with little detail.

PEER-CENTERED EXPERIENCES

Small- and Large-Group Mobility Seminars

Many educators believe that the best teachers are often the students themselves. Since the traditional mobility class is taught with a student-instructor ratio of one to one, few administrators consider assigning mobility "classes" per se. The mobility seminar is one approach to using peer counseling to reinforce learned techniques and to discuss issues and special situations in a constructive manner. Seminars can be developed with as few as two students or as many as 25. Instructors may keep the seminars tightly constructed or loosely framed, as the situations warrant. Typical discussions may center on a particular skill, for example, how to determine when you have come to a T-intersection, or on an unusual situation, such as how to handle a well-intentioned pedestrian who wishes to follow you to make sure you will not get hurt.

The seminars can be arranged to accommodate students at the same level of travel or students with various levels of skills. Instructors may wish to group students with similar skills to discuss skills and issues that are relevant to them. At other times, they may wish to group students with various levels of skills so the newer students may see students at more advanced levels.

One of the advantages of developing these seminars is to allow students to help each other solve problems. One student may be having difficulty keeping her hand centered when using the two-point-touch technique, and another student may be able to tell her how she has overcome the same problem. A second advantage is to discuss issues that have either come up during lessons or that have not yet come up but that students may be concerned about. Such topics include persistent pedestrian helpers, inaccurate information from passersby, self-defense, what one should do when the cane or cane tip breaks while traveling, how to map out an extensive area oneself, subway travel, rural travel, and breaking the mobility bonds of loved ones at home.

Mobility seminars can be an invaluable teaching and learning tool. Often, they are as important as the individual mobility lesson. Therefore, instructors must explain the importance of these lessons to their supervisors so the lessons can be incorporated into each student's mobility curriculum, when feasible.

Concept Classes, Life-Skills Classes, and Multisensory Concept Seminars

Many children and adults have difficulty understanding various concepts related to O&M. Concept classes are one means of teaching these skills. The classes are easiest to arrange in agency or institutional settings where a number of students are congregated on a regular basis. At schools for the blind, concept classes may be arranged by grouping students of similar ages and life experiences. Children of preschool age may be involved in activities (such as games like Simon Says, Red Light/Green Light, Mother May I? and the Hokey Poky) that are centered on learning body parts and spatial awareness. Later, they may learn about clocks (as referents for cardinal directions, crossing intersections "clockwise" and "counterclockwise," and so forth), landmarks, cardinal directions, and the like.

Older students can be involved in life-skills classes in which they receive transitional experiences to work and independent living situations. They may not only learn how to travel in advanced commercial environments, but they can use their travel abilities to set up bank accounts; shop for groceries; look for apartments and shop for furniture and other household goods; use public transportation systems, including taxis, buses, and airplanes; and seek recreational facilities, such as fitness centers, theaters, bowling alleys, parks, civic centers, libraries, and sports complexes.

On the other hand, adults who did not receive O&M instruction at an earlier age and hence may have gaps in their knowledge of certain spatial concepts may attend multisensory concept seminars. At some agencies for the blind, these weekly seminars have been arranged to group students of various levels of skills to learn (or relearn) linear and other spatial and environmental concepts, as detailed in Chapter 2. Understanding the concepts of "points" and "straight lines" to hear and walk straight-line routes and learning how to visualize the configurations of various floors of a building without actually being on those floors (and being able to point to the approximate location of objects outside a particular room or on different floors) are just two of the general concepts that may be taught in these seminars. Adult concept seminars must be competency based without being demeaning to the students. That is, they must revolve around activities that are appropriate to the ages of the individuals—regardless of the individuals' intellectual or experiential levels.

WORKING WITH MORE THAN ONE STUDENT AT A TIME

As was already mentioned, the usual mobility class involves one student and one instructor, but this has not always been the case. In the 1950s and 1960s, many instructors taught two or more students at a time. Several students were given a route or routes and sent off at once. It became apparent that the instructors could not do a satisfactory job of monitoring their students' safety, especially in hazardous travel situations. Over the years, it has become the accepted practice to keep the ratio to one to one to ensure student safety. However, as is the case with the mobility seminar, there are times when it is acceptable to "instruct" more than one student at a time. Another example is when the instructor assigns an independent study lesson or solo lesson to one or more students when she is physically with another student. Some students may need more time to practice their skills. If the instructor thinks that a student has learned a particular skill, she may allot time during the day for him to practice independently. The instructor may actually be working with one student outdoors while another is practicing cane skills indoors and a third student is listening to an audiotape describing an area. After the lesson period, the student or students who were working alone may briefly touch base with their instructor to provide feedback or to obtain information on problems they have encountered. This extra mobility time may be essential to give students the opportunity to have structured learning experiences and practice times during the regular workday. Although administratively it appears that the instructor is working with more than one student at a time, in reality this is not the case. If the students are not able to monitor themselves during these independent lessons, instructors may assign a mobility assistant to monitor the lessons and to reinforce the skills.

INVOLVING OTHERS IN THE LESSONS

Because the mobility instructor can be with her student only for brief periods during the day or week, it is necessary for others to be involved in the lessons, to varying degrees, to ensure consistency and continuity between formal lessons. No matter what the setting, others play an important role in the learning process. If students do not use their skills in real and normal situations, all the instruction, time, and effort will have gone for naught.

The instructor must assess who the significant members of the student's life are, depending on the setting and situation. For example, if the student lives at a school for the blind, his classroom teachers by day and the houseparents by night are an integral part of his educational experiences. Therefore, the O&M instructor not only informs the teachers of the skills to be reinforced during the day but teaches the houseparents the skills so they understand the importance of performing them correctly—even at night. Also, both should use the same vocabulary as is used during mobility lessons. A student at a public school may have a teacher's aide who not only helps him with his assignments but guides him to various places throughout the school. Furthermore, other students in the school may wish to help him. Thus, the instructor shows students how to be proper sighted guides, so no one student has the sole responsibility to be the guide.

No matter who becomes involved in the lessons, it is important to include them early on in the training. The other players in the process should become involved only when the students become proficient in the skills—not beforehand. That is, students should be allowed the freedom to learn and make mistakes unencumbered by the watchful eyes of others. Once they have learned sufficiently—at the end of a particular unit of instruction—their family members or other teachers should then be allowed to observe them during a lesson. In those circumstances, O&M instructors are better able to explain what is happening in the lesson, why their students handled situations in particular ways, and how they might have handled them differently, if appropriate. This interaction gives the visitors an opportunity to see the students in successful situations, answer any questions they may have, and alleviate any fears about their travel abilities.

Instructors thus make the teachers, peers, and family members active participants in the O&M program, so they become as much a part of the mobility process as are the students. In fact, instructors consider these others as much their "students" as they do their actual students.

Depending on the skill and unit being learned, the family members or teachers can become involved in the actual lesson in a variety of ways. First, as observers they can ask questions of the instructors. Second, as "students," parents learn from their children how to be proper sighted guides. Third, as "paraprofessionals" who reinforce skills, they can learn the correct way to monitor, teach, or reinforce the basic skills during the lesson.

This chapter has explained what it means to be a conscientious O&M teacher. For every student, there are a variety of ways to introduce and reinforce skills or concepts and a variety of persons who are important to him or her in the learning process. It is up to the instructor to become aware of the options and select the appropriate ones for a particular student.

12

Professional Issues

This chapter briefly explores a number of professional issues that the O&M instructor confronts daily. These issues may be lumped together under the term *instructor's responsibilities*, or the individual's handling of them may be considered a predicate for becoming a professional. No matter how they are viewed, they are concerns of the modern-day O&M instructor. Many suggest that these issues set the mobility instructor apart from others who work with persons who have visual impairments.

CONFIDENTIALITY AND THE STUDENT-INSTRUCTOR RELATIONSHIP

In the course of an O&M program, the O&M instructor may be confronted with situations in which information about the student may arise in the course of conversations with others. It is tempting to discuss one's student with others, but often the student's personal life should not be open to scrutiny. The O&M instructor is in a unique position to develop a close professional relationship with his students. The O&M program forces the student to face her fear of travel and to become independent of others. Likewise, persons who are important to the student, whether family members, friends, or teachers, have developed close, personal bonds with her. During the course of the O&M program, these relationships can become strained as the student becomes less dependent.

Because of the unique relationship between the student and the O&M instructor, it is important for the instructor to participate in planning the student's overall curriculum. In schools, these meetings are called Individual Education Plans (IEPs), and in agencies they are called Individual Written Rehabilitation Plans (IWRPs). Unfortunately, mobility is often considered a "related service" in schools, rather than an academic subject, so the instructor is not required to attend but may be invited. However, many times schools do not invite the O&M instructor to come to an IEP meeting because the school officials either do not know about the service or do not wish to expend school funds on O&M instruction. Hence, it is important for parents to be knowledgeable about the service and to advocate strongly for O&M instruction for their children.

Often, the O&M instructor becomes the student's confidante. The fine line must not be crossed, however, between information that is pertinent and relevant to the lessons for learning to take place and information that explores the student's personal relationships and inner feelings. The instructor must tread these waters carefully because he is not a counselor, psychologist, or social worker.

As they work together, the instructor may learn during the course of a conversation, for example, that the student is not allowed to use her cane at home but must rely on her family for sighted assistance wherever they travel. It would be tempting to call the parents and confront the problem head on. However, the instructor must consider that the information may not be entirely accurate or, at the least, one sided. If it is accurate, then what may be the ramifications of confronting the parents with their reasons (and, perhaps, fears) for not allowing their child to use her cane? What does that cane actually represent to them? Is it the possible stigma of having a blind child? Is it the possibility that the child may become independent of them? Or is it all these and, in addition, other things? In any event, a confrontation may only exacerbate the problem and alienate the parents from the instructor and the instruction.

One solution to this problem may be to invite the parents to observe an O&M lesson in which they can see their child handling travel situations confidently and safely. At this time, they will be able to ask questions that have been of concern to them. Handling the problem in this manner allows the instructor to help the parents confront their own fears. They see that the child is becoming more of a complete individual. The cane, then, becomes a tool for independence, rather than a symbol of blindness.

In a different example, the student confides in her instructor that she has difficulty sleeping at night because her mother, a single parent, is entertaining in the house until the early morning hours. Although this situation is definitely affecting the O&M lessons, the instructor must be careful not to intrude into the private affairs of the family. It would be prudent in this case for the instructor to talk to the assigned school social worker. Since the situation is affecting the student's performance of lessons, the instructor cannot view the information as being outside his sphere of responsibility. Once it is learned, it should be shared with the appropriate personnel who can pursue it further.

Many times, schools and agencies have periodic staff meetings on particular students or clients. During these meetings, it would be appropriate to share information of the nature just described as long as it is done in a productive manner— solicit opinions and strategies to resolve the problem. Unfortunately, such staff meetings frequently are used to criticize students or to share stories on how difficult the students are to teach. However cathartic this may be for the instructors, it is counterproductive and betrays the student's confidentiality.

Another source of potential betrayal of the student's confidentiality is the teacher's lounge or joint office area. In this relaxed atmosphere, teachers and O&M instructors often share information learned during the course of the day or discuss personal feelings about their students. However, such discussions should be avoided at all costs. A good rule of thumb to remember is this: If it doesn't help the student learn, don't discuss it with others.

CERTIFICATION AND A CODE OF ETHICS

These examples illustrate a few of the ethical issues and considerations the instructor is confronted with almost on a daily basis. As the O&M profession matured in the mid-to-late 1960s, instructors began to recognize the need to develop minimum standards for teaching O&M to persons who were blind or visually impaired. Those instructors who were members of Interest Group IX (Orientation and Mobility) of the American Association of Workers for the Blind (AAWB), an international association of professionals working with persons with visual impairments, met to discuss and develop standards for certification. After years of meetings, such standards were ratified and adopted by the interest group and the association.

Today, these standards have been refined to reflect minimal competencies needed to teach the skills to a variety of students or clients who are blind or visually impaired or those who have other impairments in addition to visual impairments. Certification standards are an attempt to ensure consistent instruction, regardless of where instructors received their training. If instructors are asked to perform duties contrary to their professional ethics, they may cite these standards and call on their fellow certified professionals and professional association for assistance in resolving the conflict.

Certification begins with formalized instruction and training. It has become an accepted practice that persons who perform the full range of duties required of O&M instructors receive their specialized training at colleges and universities that are recognized by AER, the successor organization to the merger of AAWB and its sister association, the Association for Education of the Visually Handicapped. These institutions are recognized for providing an acceptable mobility curriculum taught by certified and experienced mobility faculty. A current listing of these universities may be found in the Resource section.

Students receive instruction in the theories of motor and sensory development, the medical aspects of blindness and associated disabilities, the psychological aspects of blindness, research theory, the methodology of teaching O&M, and supervised practice in teaching O&M to persons with visual impairments. They can either receive bachelor's or master's degrees with a specialty in O&M, or they can enroll in additional O&M courses after they receive their degrees. In either case, they then apply to AER for national certification. Mobility assistants, who perform only basic skills training, may be formally trained at a school or agency by an O&M instructor who is certified to provide this special training and the necessary ongoing supervision. These assistants may also apply for AER certification to recognize their limited expertise.

As O&M instruction has been introduced throughout the world, more and more countries are recognizing and adopting AER's standards. Over 1,300 current members of AER's Division IX (Orientation and Mobility) worldwide have endorsed these standards.

THE O&M CODE OF ETHICS

Since the early 1970s, the O&M profession has required its members who seek certification to agree to abide by a code of ethics specifically applied to teaching O&M. The code speaks to issues related to teaching O&M to the individual with a visual impairment, working in an agency or school, working in the community, and working with other professionals. The code of ethics recognizes the unique relationship between the instructor and student and provides standards and safeguards for the student. It also protects the instructor from situations that may compromise his professional opinion. The code of ethics is under continuous scrutiny and review and is modified when situations warrant.

Certification standards and a code of ethics are attempts to protect persons with visual impairments from unsafe practices and to protect instructors from knowingly placing their students in situations that compromise their judgments. Without these safeguards, anyone could and would attempt to teach O&M. Because the skills to teach O&M are varied, complex, and, in some situations, potentially dangerous and because the student's psychological and physical make-up are equally diversified and complex, it is important that well-trained individuals are allowed to teach in a way they deem professionally appropriate.

As long as the profession has members who take their responsibilities seriously, these safeguards will remain in place. It is up to these professionals to be actively involved in their professional association to ensure consistent and high-quality instruction in the future. Students in university programs are introduced to their professional association during their course of study and are encouraged to become student members of Division IX and full and contributing members of their profession and of AER after they graduate.

INSTRUCTOR'S RESPONSIBILITY AND ACKNOWLEDGMENT OF RISKS

The teaching of O&M is a holistic approach to helping the individual with a visual impairment gain security and confidence in handling all travel situations safely. Often it entails a bond of mutual trust between the instructor and student, as was mentioned earlier in this chapter. The instructor has a responsibility to analyze a student's current level of skills, develop meaningful and appropriate lessons to teach the skills, overcome the student's deficits in certain areas, and prepare the student to handle problems in appropriate ways. This process leads the student to become the best traveler that she can be.

The student must learn to trust the instructor's judgments and abilities as a teacher. As she matures from one who has been dependent on others to one who takes control over her own travel needs, the emotional and other bonds between the instructor and student should be severed.

During this process, the possibility that the student will make mistakes and be injured increases. The O&M instructor accepts these risks as part of his practice but does everything in his power to lessen the likelihood of injury to his student. He expects from his student only what the student has learned; that is, if the student gets into a situation that she has not yet experienced during lessons and has not yet learned how to handle, the instructor does not expect her to handle appropriately. As a consequence, the instructor is more likely to be physically close to the student and to intervene and use the situation as a learning experience. The next time a similar situation occurs, he may expect the student to begin handling it more appropriately and thus may stay farther away from her.

Eventually, the student should learn to take responsibility for her actions and accept the responsibility for her decisions. For example, when attempting to cross a street in the downtown unit of instruction, the student may misinterpret the sounds of the cars on the perpendicular as being those of cars on the parallel street and may begin to cross the street. The instructor may be observing several blocks away and not be in a position to come to her aid. By the nature of his physical location, the instructor trusts that the student has the skills to handle the situation in an appropriate manner, as she has done many other times when the instructor has been closer at hand. By physically widening the distance between him and the student, the instructor demonstrates his trust in his student's skills, judgments, and problem-solving abilities. The student acknowledges her responsibility in that situation by attempting to meet the objectives of the lesson that the instructor outlined to her at the start of the lesson and by the consistent skills she has shown to that point. This physical distance is critical not only for building confidence and trust, but for allowing the public to interact with the student in typical ways so she learns how to handle passersby appropriately.

LIFELONG LEARNING AND SHARING ONE'S EXPERTISE

As a professional, the O&M instructor knows that he does not teach in a vacuum but is part of the education and rehabilitation team composed of other professionals. Likewise, he knows that as he instructs his students, he is constantly learning and devising news ways to teach similar skills to persons with different cultural and educational backgrounds and levels of ability. Consequently, every instructor must learn to recognize that he has much to offer fellow professionals. This sharing of expertise and experiences can be done through in-service workshops at a school or agency or through periodic meetings to discuss pertinent issues or skills.

Membership in Professional Associations

One avenue for sharing information is through maintaining membership in one's professional association. By becoming an active member in one's professional association, one has a venue for sharing information with others and for learning from others. The O&M instructor has a professional responsibility to maintain the level of his teaching skills and to obtain state-of-the-art information related to his profession. By attending local, state, regional, and national conferences and workshops, the professional O&M instructor ensures that he gains the most current training and information that can be applied to working with his students. Usually, membership in a professional association has numerous benefits: interactions with fellow professionals; leadership in influencing the direction of the profession; access to professional journals and newsletters; and access to life, health, disability, and liability insurance, to name a few.

Writing for Publication

As long as the O&M instructor remains in his profession, he recognizes his professional responsibility to maintain his teaching competence and to share his knowledge with colleagues. He can do so by writing for publication in professional journals. Unfortunately, many instructors do not avail themselves of this opportunity for fear that they do not have adequate writing skills or the time to write. By writing for professional journals, the O&M instructor recognizes that he has something to share and is willing to expose his ideas to discussion and debate. New ideas thoughtfully expressed are not easily accepted by others. However, without them, the profession remains stagnant and does not grow. Furthermore, by writing and sharing ideas, the instructor contributes to the growth of the profession and ensures that future professionals (and their students) will learn from both his successful and unsuccessful teaching experiences.

PURSUING ADVANCED DEGREES AND LEADERSHIP POSITIONS

Others in the profession recognize the importance of exploring new research ideas in formal ways. Through doctoral programs, future leaders emerge. It is hoped that those who choose this direction will become faculty members at university O&M programs. Without the infusion of doctoral-level personnel in university O&M programs, the very survival of these programs (and, ultimately, of the profession) will be at risk.

Finally, many who decide to become O&M instructors find themselves thrust into positions of additional authority and responsibility. Some become supervisors or administrators. These leaders will direct the future of educational and rehabilitation services for persons with visual impairments.

Whatever one's future goals, the profession of O&M demands personal growth and development. This is a responsibility that one cannot ignore and remain a truly involved member of the O&M profession.

References

Allen, W., Griffith, A., & Shaw, C. (1977). *Orientation and mobility: Behavioral objectives for teaching older adventitiously blind individuals*. New York: New York Infirmary/Center for Independent Living.

Cratty, B. J., & Sams, T. A. (July, 1968). *The body image of blind children* (Research Bulletin No. 17). New York: American Foundation for the Blind.

Croce, R. V., & Jacobson, W. H. (1986). The application of two point touch cane technique to theories of motor control and learning: Implications for orientation and mobility training. *Journal of Visual Impairment & Blindness, 80*, 790-793.

Dauterman, W. L. (1972). *Manual for the Stanford Multi-Modality Imagery Test*. New York: American Foundation for the Blind.

Edman, P. K. (1992). *Tactile graphics*. New York: American Foundation for the Blind.

Fraiberg, S., Smith, M., & Adelson, E. (1969). An educational program for blind infants. *Journal of Special Education, 3*, 121-139.

Gill, J. M. (Ed.) (in press). *Equipment for visually disabled people: An international guide*. London, England: Royal National Institute for the Blind.

Hill, E. W. (1981). *Hill Performance Test on Selected Positional Concepts*. Chicago: Stoelting Co.

Hill, E. W. (1986). Orientation and mobility. In G. T. Scholl (Ed.), *Foundations of education for blind and visually handicapped children and youth: Theory and practice* (pp. 315-340). New York: American Foundation for the Blind.

Hill, E. W., & Blasch, B. B. (1980). Concept development. In R. L. Welsh & B. B. Blasch (Eds.), *Foundations of orientation and mobility* (pp. 265-290). New York: American Foundation for the Blind.

Hill, E., & Ponder, P. (1976). *Orientation and mobility techniques: A guide for the practitioner*. New York: American Foundation for the Blind.

Lord, F. E. (1969-1970). Development of scales for the measurement of orientation and mobility of young blind children. *Exceptional Children, 36*(2), 77-81.

National Society to Prevent Blindness. (1980). *Vision problems in the U.S.: A statistical analysis prepared by Operational Research Department, NSPB.* New York: Author.

Scholl, G. T. (1986). Growth and development. In G. T. Scholl (Ed.), *Foundations of education for blind and visually handicapped children and youth: Theory and practice* (pp. 65-81). New York: American Foundation for the Blind.

Uslan, M. M., Peck, A F., Wiener, W. R., & Stern, A. (Eds.). (1990). *Access to mass transit for blind and visually impaired travelers.* New York: American Foundation for the Blind.

Welsh, R. L., & Blasch, B. B. (Eds.). (1980). *Foundations of orientation and mobility.* New York: American Foundation for the Blind.

Resources

A wide variety of organizations and agencies disseminate useful information and provide assistance to people who are blind or visually impaired, their families, and the professionals who work with them. This section contains a sample list of organizations, schools, and companies that provide information, training, and products useful to individuals in the field of orientation and mobility. Additional information on these and other sources of assistance, materials, and equipment can be found in the *Directory of Services for Blind and Visually Impaired Persons in the United States and Canada, 24th Edition,* published by the American Foundation for the Blind.

SOURCES OF INFORMATION

American Council of the Blind
1155 15th Street, N.W., Suite 720
Washington, DC 20005
(202) 467-5081 or (800) 424-8666
The American Council of the Blind (ACB) is a consumer organization that promotes effective participation of blind people in all aspects of society. It provides information and referral, legal assistance, scholarships, advocacy, consultation, and program development assistance and publishes The Braille Forum.

American Foundation for the Blind
15 West 16th Street
New York, NY 10011
(212) 620-2000 or (800) 232-5463 (hotline)
The American Foundation for the Blind (AFB) provides a wide variety of services to and acts as an information clearinghouse for people who are blind or visually impaired and their families, professionals, organizations, schools, and corporations. It conducts information and educational programs; stimulates research to improve services to visually impaired persons; develops and sells adapted products; advocates for services and legislation; maintains

the M. C. Migel Memorial Library and the Helen Keller Archives; and publishes books, pamphlets, videos, the Directory of Services for Blind and Visually Impaired Persons in the United States and Canada, *and the* Journal of Visual Impairment & Blindness. *AFB maintains the following regional centers across the country, as well as a governmental relations department in Washington, DC.*

Eastern Regional Center
1615 M Street, N.W., Suite 250
Washington, DC 20036
(202) 457-1487
Serves Connecticut, Delaware, District of Columbia, Maine, Maryland, Massachusetts, New Hampshire, New Jersey, New York, Pennsylvania, Rhode Island, Vermont, and Virginia.

Midwest Regional Center
401 North Michigan Avenue, Suite 308
Chicago, IL 60611
(312) 245-9961
Serves Illinois, Indiana, Iowa, Kentucky, Michigan, Minnesota, Missouri, North Dakota, Ohio, South Dakota, and Wisconsin.

Southeast Regional Center
100 Peachtree Street, Suite 620
Atlanta, GA 30303
(404) 525-2303
Serves Alabama, Florida, Georgia, Mississippi, North Carolina, Puerto Rico, South Carolina, Tennessee, the Virgin Islands, and West Virginia.

Southwest Regional Center
260 Treadway Plaza
Exchange Park
Dallas, TX 75235
(214) 352-7222
Serves Arkansas, Colorado, Kansas, Louisiana, Montana, Nebraska, New Mexico, Oklahoma, Texas, and Wyoming.

Western Regional Center
111 Pine Street, Suite 725
San Francisco, CA 94111
(415) 392-4845
Serves Alaska, Arizona, California, Guam, Hawaii, Idaho, Nevada, Oregon, Utah, and Washington.

American Printing House for the Blind
1839 Frankfort Avenue
P.O. Box 6085
Louisville, KY 40206-0085
(502) 895-2405 or (800) 223-1839
The American Printing House for the Blind (APH) administers an annual appropriation from Congress to provide textbooks and educational aids for legally blind students. It also produces materials in braille and large print and on audiocassette; manufactures computer-access equipment, software, and special educational devices for visually impaired persons; and maintains an educational research and development program and a reference-catalog service.

Association for Education and Rehabilitation of the Blind and Visually Impaired
Division IX (Orientation and Mobility)
206 North Washington Street, Suite 320
Alexandria, VA 22314
(703) 548-1884
The Association for Education and Rehabilitation of the Blind and Visually Impaired (AER) is a professional membership organization that promotes all phases of education and work for blind and visually impaired persons of all ages, strives to expand their opportunities to take a contributory place in society, and disseminates information. It also certifies rehabilitation teachers, orientation and mobility specialists, and classroom teachers and publishes RE:view, AER Report, *and* Job Exchange Monthly.

Canadian National Institute for the Blind
1929 Bayview Avenue
Toronto, Ontario M4G 3E8
Canada
(416) 486-2500
The Canadian National Institute for the Blind (CNIB) provides a wide variety of services to persons who are blind or visually impaired, including orientation and mobility training, counseling, and rehabilitation teaching.

Council for Exceptional Children
1920 Association Drive
Reston, VA 22091-1589
(703) 620-3660
The Council for Exceptional Children (CEC) is a professional organization for teachers, administrators, and others who are concerned with children who require special services. It publishes position papers as well as periodicals, books, and other materials on teaching exceptional children.

Council of U.S. Guide Dog Schools
c/o Guiding Eyes for the Blind
611 Granite Springs Road
Yorktown Heights, NY 10598
(914) 245-4024
The Council of U.S. Guide Dog Schools provides consultation on dog guides and dog guide schools.

Helen Keller International
90 Washington Street
New York, NY 10006
(212) 943-0890
Helen Keller International (HKI) provides consultation and assistance to developing nations to help them establish programs to prevent blindness and to educate or rehabilitate blind children and adults.

Helen Keller National Center for Deaf-Blind Youths and Adults
111 Middle Neck Road
Sands Point, NY 11050
(516) 944-8900
The Helen Keller National Center for Deaf-Blind Youths and Adults provides technical assistance to facilitate the transition of deaf-blind youths from educational services to community-based adult services.

National Accreditation Council of State Agencies for the Blind
15 East 40th Street, Suite 1004
New York, NY 10016
(212) 683-5068
The National Accreditation Council of State Agencies for the Blind (NAC) oversees the accreditation of programs, agencies, and schools serving blind and visually impaired persons.

National Association for Parents of the Visually Impaired
P.O. Box 317
Watertown, MA 02272-0317
(800) 562-6265
The National Association for Parents of the Visually Impaired (NAPVI) is a consumer membership organization for parents of visually impaired children. It operates a national clearinghouse of information, supports parents' groups and workshops across the United States, and publishes the newsletter Awareness.

National Federation of the Blind
1800 Johnson Street
Baltimore, MD 21230
(410) 659-9314
The National Federation of the Blind (NFB) is a consumer organization that strives to improve social and economic conditions of blind persons, evaluates and assists in establishing programs, and provides public education and scholarships. It also publishes The Braille Monitor *and* Future Reflections.

National Rehabilitation Association
633 South Washington Street
Alexandria, VA 22314
(703) 836-0850
The National Rehabilitation Association is a professional organization that provides consultation on issues related to disability and publishes journals and other materials.

Royal National Institute for the Blind
Technical Development Department
224 Great Portland Street
London W1N 6AA
England
44-21-643-9912
The Royal National Institute for the Blind (RNIB) conducts research, publishes directories of international research in blindness, and supplies equipment for persons with visual impairments to an international market.

U.S. Department of Education
330 C Street, S.W.
Washington, DC 20202
(202) 205-9316
The U.S. Department of Education administers a wide variety of programs and procedures relating to people who are blind or visually impaired. The Office of Special Education and Rehabilitative Services (OSERS), (202) 205-5465, oversees federal personnel preparation programs and special education policies. The Office of Special Education Programs, (202) 205-5507, administers the Individuals with Disabilities Education Act and related pro-

grams for the education of children with disabilities. The Rehabilitation Services Administration (RSA), (202) 205-5482, administers grants and oversees programs related to the vocational rehabilitation of blind and visually impaired persons.

U.S. Department of Veterans Affairs
Blind Rehabilitation Service
810 Vermont Avenue, N.W.
Washington, DC 20420
(202) 535-7637
The U.S. Department of Veterans Affairs provides a wide variety of services, including orientation and mobility instruction, to blinded U.S. military veterans.

ORIENTATION AND MOBILITY PREPARATION PROGRAMS*†

Australia
La Trobe University
Department of Behavioural Services
Bundoora Campus
Plenty Road
Bundoora 3083
Australia
03-479-1750

Belgium
IRSA
Chaussu de Waterloo, 1504
1180 Bruxelles
Belgium
32-2-374-9090, ext. 255

Koninklijk Institute Spermalie
Snaggaardstraat 9
B-8000 Bruges
Belgium
32-150-340-341

Canada
Mohawk College of Applied Arts and Technology
Brant Campuses
411 Elgin Street
Brantford, Ontario N3T 5V2
Canada
(519) 758-6043

---

*Programs currently endorsed by Division IX (Orientation and Mobility) of the Association for Education and Rehabilitation of the Blind and Visually Impaired.
†Programs undergoing (or soon to be undergoing) endorsement by Division IX (Orientation and Mobility) of the Association for Education and Rehabilitation of the Blind and Visually Impaired.

University of British Columbia
Education Psychology and Special Education Department
Vancouver, British Columbia V6T 1Z4
Canada
(604) 822-5538

University of Sherbrooke
Faculty of Education
Sherbrooke, Quebec J1K 2R1
Canada
(819) 821-7438

Germany
Ausbildungsstatte fur Rehabilitationslehrer fur Blinde und Sehbehinderte
Am Schlag 8
D-3550 Marburg 1
Germany
49-6421-606-173 or 49-6421-606-174

Deutsche Blindenstudienstalt
Postfach 1160
D-3550 Marburg
Germany
49-6421-606-773

Institute for Rehabilitation and Integration of the Sight Impaired
Sierichstrasse 56
D-2000 Hamburg 60
Germany
49-40-270-0422

Padogogische Hochschule
6900 Heidelberg
Germany
49-6221-477-410 or 49-6221-477-400

Ghana
National Mobility Centre
Accra 227101
Ghana

Israel
Migdal Or (American Israeli Lighthouse)
Rehabilitation Teachers Division
Kiriat Haim
Israel

Japan
Research Institute
National Rehabilitation Center for the Disabled
1, 4-chome, Namiki
Tokorozawa, Saitama 359

Japan
81-429-95-3100

Netherlands

Dutch Association for the Blind and Partially Sighted People
Utrecht
The Netherlands
31-30-443-336

Stichting Revalidate van Blinde en Slechtziende Volwassenen
Waldeck Pyrmonstraat 31
7315 JH Apeldoorn
The Netherlands

Theofaan Institut voor Blinden en Slechtzienden
St. Elizabethstraat 4
5361 HK Grave
The Netherlands
31-8860-71003 or 31-8860-75919

New Zealand

Massey University*
Rehabilitation Studies Section
Department of Psychology
Palmerston North
New Zealand
64-63-69-099

Spain

La Laguna University
Didactic and Educational and Behavioral Research Department
La Laguna, Tenerife, Canary Islands
Spain
34-922-220-303

ONCE (Organization Nacional de Ciegos Espagnoles)
Calle del Prado 24
28104 Madrid
Spain
34-1-429-9642

United Kingdom

Royal National Institute for the Blind
224 Great Portland Street
London, W1N 6AA
England
44-21-643-9912

United States

ARIZONA
University of Arizona[†]
College of Education

Department of Special Education
Tucson, AZ 85721
(602) 621-7822

ARKANSAS
University of Arkansas at Little Rock*
Department of Rehabilitation
2801 South University Avenue
Little Rock, AR 72204
(501) 569-3169

CALIFORNIA
California State University at Los Angeles*
Department of Special Education
5151 State University Drive
Los Angeles, CA 90032
(213) 343-4411

San Francisco State University*
Department of Special Education
1600 Holloway Avenue
San Francisco, CA 94132
(415) 338-1080

COLORADO
University of Northern Colorado*
Division of Special Education
Greeley, CO 80639
(303) 351-2691

FLORIDA
Florida State University*
College of Education
Visual Impairments B-172
Tallahassee, FL 32306
(904) 644-4880

ILLINOIS
Northern Illinois University*
Department of Learning, Development, and Special Education
Dekalb, IL 60115
(815) 753-8459

MASSACHUSETTS
University of Massachusetts at Boston†
Graduate College of Education
Harbor Campus
Boston, MA 02125-3393
(617) 287-5709

MICHIGAN
Michigan State University*
Department of Counseling, Educational Psychology

331 Erickson Hall
East Lansing, MI 48824
(517) 355-1871

Western Michigan University*
Department of Blind Rehabilitation
Kalamazoo, MI 49008
(616) 387-3455

PENNSYLVANIA
Pennsylvania College of Optometry*
Institute for the Visually Impaired
Department of Graduate Studies in Vision Impairment
1200 West Godfrey Avenue
Philadelphia, PA 19141
(215) 276-6292

University of Pittsburgh*
School of Education
Department of Special Education
4H01 Forbes Quadrangle
Pittsburgh, PA 15260
(412) 624-7254

SOUTH CAROLINA
South Carolina State College†
Department of Human Services/Rehabilitation Counseling
300 College Street, N.E.
Orangeburg, SC 20117-0001
(803) 536-8889

TENNESSEE
George Peabody College for Teachers*
Vanderbilt University
Department of Special Education
Box 328
Nashville, TN 37203
(615) 322-8160

TEXAS
Stephen F. Austin State University*
SFA Station, Box 13019
Nacogdoches, TX 75962
(409) 568-2906

Texas Tech University*
College of Education
Box 41071
Lubbock, TX 79409-1071
(806) 742-2320 or (806) 742-2345

University of Texas at Austin*
College of Education, Building 306

Department of Special Education
Austin, TX 78712-1290
(512) 471-4161

SOURCES OF LONG CANES
AmbuTech
670 Golspie Street
Winnipeg, Ontario R2K 2V1
Canada
(800) 561-3340 (continental United States only)
Types available: AmbuTech folding mobility cane with marshmallow tip, folding identification cane. Cane repair and refurbishing services are also available.

American Foundation for the Blind (AFB)
15 West 16th Street
New York, NY 10011
(212) 620-2000 or (800) 829-0500 (United States) or (302) 677-0200 (international)
Types available: AFB Superfold cane, AFB Kiddy cane, Mahler folding and rigid canes.

Autofold, Inc.
P.O. Box 1063
208 Coleman Street
Gardner, MA 01440-1063
(508) 632-0667
Types available: Autofold cane, Autofold Delux cane (double cord, extra tip), rigid fiberglass cane with crook handle, Cable cane, High Fashion Low Vision walking stick, white tactile rigid cane (length, 56").

Cape Town Civilian Blind Society
45 Salt River Road
Salt River 7925
Republic of South Africa
Types available: Bundu Basher cane, Bundu tips.

Independent Living Aids, Inc.
27 East Mall
Plainview, NY 11803
(516) 752-8080 or (800) 537-2118
Types available: White Cane Instruments for the Blind (WCIB) canes, Mahler canes.

LS&S Group, Inc.
P.O. Box 673
Northbrook, IL 60065
(708) 498-9777 or (800) 468-4789
Types available: AmbuTech folding cane with marshmallow tip, AmbuTech identification cane, WCIB cane with golf grip, WCIB rigid cane with golf grip, WCIB rigid cane with crook, LS&S heavy-duty folding cane (1/2" aluminum tubing), heavy-duty Mahler folding cane.

Macam Devices
774 Hamlin Way
San Leandro, CA 94578

(415) 582-1878
Types available: Equipoise long cane.

Maxi-Aids
P.O. Box 3209
Farmingdale, NY 11735
(516) 752-0521 or (800) 522-6294
Types available: Europa folding aluminum cane with golf grip, Europa rigid fiberglass cane with golf grip, Maxi Superior folding cane, Mahler Superior folding cane, WCIB heavy-duty folding cane, Maxi Lite folding cane, fiberglass cane, wooden cane (can be cut to specifications, length: 42" with metal glide tip), telescopic aluminum cane, rigid aluminum cane with crook.

Mobility Services, Inc.
761 Peachtree Street, N.E.
Atlanta, GA 30308
(404) 876-2636 or (800) 876-2636
Types available: Mobility long canes with golf, ambidextrous grip, Autofold cane with bicycle and golf grips.

National Federation of the Blind (NFB)
1800 Johnson Street
Baltimore, MD 21230
(301) 659-9314
Types available: NFB long cane and folding cane.

Royal National Institute for the Blind
Technical Development Department
224 Great Portland Street
London W1N 6AA
England
A variety of aids and appliances for persons with visual impairments are available. Equipment for Visually Disabled People: An International Guide, *a listing of international manufacturers of canes and other equipment, is also available.*

Sense-Sations
919 Walnut Street
Philadelphia, PA 19107
(215) 627-0600
Types available: WCIB folding and rigid canes, Hycor folding cane, Mahler folding cane.

VisAids, Inc.
102-08 Jamaica Avenue
Richmond Hill, NY 11418
(800) 346-9579
Types available: Mahler heavy-duty folding cane with golf grip, WCIB heavy-duty folding cane, VisAids Lite folding cane, VisAids Superior folding cane, telescopic aluminum cane (44"-56").

White Cane Instruments for the Blind (WCIB)
Route 3

Jenkins, MO 65605
(417) 574-6368
Types available: WCIB rigid cane, WCIB folding cane.

SOURCES OF ELECTRONIC TRAVEL AIDS

Brytech
28 Concourse Gate, Suite 102
Nepean, Ontario K2E 7T7
Canada
(613) 727-5800
Types available: Sensory 6, an ultrasonic mobility device.

HumanWare
6245 King Road
Loomis, CA 95650
(916) 652-7253 or (800) 722-3393
Types available: Mowat Sensor, Sonicguide.

Mobility Services, Inc.
761 Peachtree Street, N.E.
Atlanta, GA 30308
(404) 876-2636 or (800) 876-2636
Types available: Mowat Sensor.

Nurion Industries
Station Square Three
Paoli, PA 19301
(215) 640-22345
Types available: Laser cane, Polaron, Wheelchair Pathfinder.

Pulse Data International, Ltd.
P.O. Box 3044
Christchurch
New Zealand
64-3-794-011
Types available: Mowat Sensor.

Index

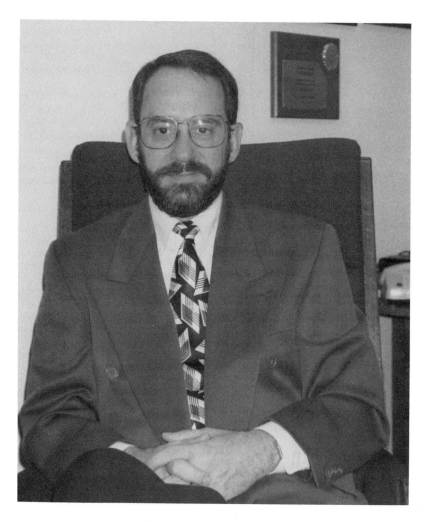

About the Author

William H. Jacobson is professor of rehabilitation of the blind, University of Arkansas at Little Rock, and has coordinated the orientation and mobility (O&M) program since 1981. Previously, he taught O&M to children and adults with visual impairments at the Atlanta public schools and Community Services for the Blind in Atlanta, Georgia, and at the Northeastern Rehabilitation Center for the Blind in Albany, New York. He received a bachelor's degree in education with an emphasis in special education—teaching the visually handicapped child—from Ohio State University, a master's degree in peripatology from Boston College, and a doctoral degree in special education and public administration from the University of Arkansas, Fayetteville. He has written numerous articles on O&M for such publications as the *Journal of Visual Impairment and Blindness* and *Review of Optometry* and served as chairperson of Division IX (Orientation and Mobility) of the Association for Education and Rehabilitation of the Blind and Visually Impaired, 1992-94.